Noor Nadheer Al-Taie
Shaho Ziyad Al-Talabani

Perception and Awareness Towards Dental Artificial Intelligence

Noor Nadheer Al-Taie
Shaho Ziyad Al-Talabani

Perception and Awareness Towards Dental Artificial Intelligence

in Orthodontic Practice Among Iraqi Orthodontists

LAP LAMBERT Academic Publishing

Imprint
Any brand names and product names mentioned in this book are subject to trademark, brand or patent protection and are trademarks or registered trademarks of their respective holders. The use of brand names, product names, common names, trade names, product descriptions etc. even without a particular marking in this work is in no way to be construed to mean that such names may be regarded as unrestricted in respect of trademark and brand protection legislation and could thus be used by anyone.

Cover image: www.ingimage.com

Publisher:
LAP LAMBERT Academic Publishing
is a trademark of
Dodo Books Indian Ocean Ltd. and OmniScriptum S.R.L publishing group

120 High Road, East Finchley, London, N2 9ED, United Kingdom
Str. Armeneasca 28/1, office 1, Chisinau MD-2012, Republic of Moldova, Europe
Managing Directors: Ieva Konstantinova, Victoria Ursu
info@omniscriptum.com

Printed at: see last page
ISBN: 978-620-9-41456-5

DEDICATION

All praise and gratitude be to Allah, who enlightened my heart and guided my steps, praise befitting His Majesty and Greatness.

This journey, with all its late nights, quiet battles, tireless efforts, and every word my pen poured into the pages of this thesis, is lovingly dedicated:

To the unwavering pillars of my life—my beloved parents, my shelter, and my strength.

To the heartbeat of my soul and the light of my life, my dearest siblings.

To every soul who supported, encouraged, or uplifted me, even with a single word.

To all of you, I dedicate this humble achievement.

Noor Nadheer Al-Taie

ACKNOWLEDGMENTS

With the deepest gratitude, I first and foremost thank ALLAH, the Most Gracious, the Most Merciful, whose light guided me through every step of this academic journey. I owe my heartfelt gratitude to my beloved family, whose boundless love and encouragement have been the silent force behind it all.

My profound gratitude goes to my supervisor, Assistant Professor Dr. Shaho Ziyad Jamil, for his patient mentorship, thoughtful guidance, and unwavering support. His openness to my academic inquiries and scientific curiosity played a vital role in shaping this research.

Special appreciation is extended to Dean Professor Dr. Bassam Karim Amin, whose dedication and commitment have significantly contributed to the college's academic progress.

Special thanks and sincere appreciation go to the Head of the Orthodontic Department, Dr. Brwa Mahdi Khoshnaw, and to my esteemed mentors in the postgraduate program, Dr.Zana Qadir Omar, Dr. Omar Fawzi Chawshli, and Dr. Bayan Abdulla Hassan, for their support and guidance throughout both the academic and clinical stages of my master's journey.

I am also deeply grateful to the expert panel members from the Universities of Baghdad, Mosul, Sulaimaniyah, and Hawler Medical University, whose valuable feedback and active participation in developing and validating this study greatly enhanced its academic rigor.

My sincere thanks go to the President and members of the Iraqi Orthodontic Society for their kind cooperation and valuable participation, which enriched this research with essential perspectives and meaningful data.

I wish to express my deepest appreciation to Hiba Bookstore and its proprietor, Mr. Lame', for his substantial support and gracious assistance throughout this academic experience.

Finally, I want to sincerely thank my dear and loyal colleagues. To everyone who stood beside me—whether in silence, speech, presence, or prayer-thank you from the bottom of my heart.

ABSTRACT

Background and Objectives: The use of artificial intelligence is rapidly expanding and has had a significant impact on the orthodontic domain. Designing a validated survey study to investigate the knowledge and attitudes of specialized orthodontists regarding the application of artificial intelligence in orthodontic practice was the goal of this study.

Methods: An anonymous, web-based cross-sectional study was performed among orthodontists in Iraq applying the Google Forms platform. The survey instrument was evaluated by an expert panel for content validity using Lawshe's method and for face validity by measuring inter-rater reliability. The survey included “25 closed-ended and one open-ended question” organized into six sections. After its official release, the survey link was disseminated to all Iraqi Orthodontic Society members from January to March 2025. Descriptive statistics were conducted to categorize the respondents' age groups.

Results: One hundred and one valid surveys were collected and analyzed, highlighting a 63% response rate. The results pointed out that although a significant proportion of respondents (61.4%) recognized the utilization of AI-driven software in orthodontics, a considerable percentage (40.6%) reported that they had never used such programs, underscoring a certain level of deficiency in the implementation of artificial intelligence in orthodontic practice. The awareness level was higher for artificial intelligence applications in cephalometric analysis (60.0%) compared to other applications, such as orthognathic surgery and the biomechanics domain. Most participants (95.0%) strongly recommended integrating AI-related training into undergraduate and postgraduate orthodontic curricula.

Conclusion: Overall, there was a good level of awareness and knowledge regarding AI's role in orthodontics, with strong readiness among the specialists to participate in AI-related training and integrate it into their clinical routines. The study supports further education, training, evidence-based validation, and designing more AI-powered tools addressing different domains of orthodontics, particularly biomechanics, which are essential to bridge the trust gap. Orthodontists should be encouraged to adopt AI as a supportive tool while prioritizing patients' well-being as the foremost priority in clinical decision-making.

Keywords: Artificial intelligence, Attitudes of health personnel, Clinical practice, Knowledge, Orthodontics, Perception

PUBLICATION

Al-Taie, N. N., & Al-Talabani, S. Z. (2025). Perception and Application of Dental Artificial Intelligence in Orthodontic Clinical Practice: A Cross-Sectional Survey of Orthodontists in Iraq. Al-Rafidain Journal of Medical Sciences (ISSN 2789-3219), 9(1), 39–47. Available from https://ajms.iq/index.php/ALRAFIDAIN/article/view/2050

Table of contents

List of Tables

List of Figures

List of Abbreviations

Abbreviations	Complete statement
3D	Three-dimentional
AH	Adenoid hypertrophy
AI	Artificial intelligence
ANNs	Artificial neural networks
CAD-CAM	Computer-aided design and Computer-aided technology
CBCT	Cone beam computed tomography
CKI	Cohen's kappa index
CNNs	Convolutional neural networks
CVI	Content validity index
CVM	Cervical vertebrae maturation
CVR	Content validity ratio
DICOM	Digital imaging and communications in medicine
DL	Deep learning
IOS	Iraqi Orthodontic Society
K	Kappa
MENA	Middle East and North Africa
ML	Machine learning
MSc	Master of Science
OPG	Orthopantomogram

OSA	Obstructive sleep apnea
PhD	Doctor of Philosophy
STL	Standard tessellation language
TAD	Temporary anchorage device
TMJ	Temporomandibular joint
TMJ-OA	Temporomandibular joint osteoarthritis
UCP	Unilateral cleft palate

INTRODUCTION

Artificial intelligence (AI) is an innovation that refers to the development of robots that can imitate human thinking and operate autonomously with minimal personal involvement.(Hamet and Tremblay, 2017; Mohammad-Rahimi et al., 2021)

Dental physicians have got benefit from the development of AI technology. It can analyze data in various forms, including patient history, treatment records, and demographic information, assist in determining patient priorities and individual requirements, and increase accountability and motivation for patients' health. AI-enabled intelligent assistants and chatbots can facilitate dental consultations through teledentistry. (Thorat et al., 2024)

Many branches of dentistry have benefited from AI advancements, such as radiology, periodontics, oral pathology, oral surgery, endodontics, prosthodontics, and orthodontics.(Park et al., 2021; Shan et al., 2021; Fatima et al., 2022; Miragall et al., 2023; Larkin et al., 2024).

Artificial intelligence has revolutionized orthodontics. It has been employed for facial analysis, estimating the maturation level of cervical vertebrae, digitizing and tracing cephalometric landmarks with 90% accuracy, and predicting orthodontic outcomes.(Hanenkrath et al., 2025)

Orthodontic research has investigated AI implementation in many fields, such as extraction decision-making, airway analysis, evaluating the necessity of orthognathic surgery, and estimating facial aesthetics after orthognathic surgery to enhance accuracy and avoid bias from less experienced professionals. Most AI models in this field rely primarily on artificial neural networks (ANNs) or convolutional neural networks (CNNs).(Topol, 2019; Khanagar et al., 2021a; Lin et al., 2023). Tele-orthodontics represents an innovation in remote monitoring during clear aligner therapy.(Thurzo et al., 2021)

Technological advances have further evolved, including real-time tooth modelling, three-dimensional printing, intraoral scans, robotic-assisted procedures, three-dimensional visualization, and facial scanners.(Monill-González et al., 2021). Future systems will likely be most efficient in conducting patient trials and screening independently and precisely.(Mengi et al., 2024)

While AI has great potential, its everyday use in dental practice is still limited. Challenges that impede wider adoption include data openness, non-replicability, and lack of robustness in dental artificial intelligence (AI) research and the constraints of current AI applications.(Schwendicke et al., 2020).Data confidentiality and security challenges, algorithms' limited generalizability, and built-in bias that could bias diagnostic or treatment recommendations are also points of concern.(Schwendicke et al., 2020; Pethani, 2021)

Transparency in algorithm decision-making is becoming increasingly important due to the "black-box opaque nature" of algorithm design.(Ding et al., 2023). Furthermore, excessive dependence on technology can lead to a diminished role for humans, compromising both efficiency and comprehensiveness concerning the service provided.(Thorat et al., 2024)

AI Research— exploring new frontiers for addressing issues and translating research into valuable clinical tools, including interactions between clinicians and technology personnel. It also includes evaluating the effect of these AI technologies on medical care's productivity, speed, and efficiency, as well as understanding users' approaches to adopting technologies such as AI.(TaherdoostP, 2018; Kelly et al., 2019). Acceptance and experience of users can significantly affect their attitude and perception of adopting new technology. (Rahimi et al., 2018; Taherdoost, 2018; Distler et al., 2020)

However, AI's potential is significant if these issues can be overcome. AI can optimize clinical workflows, harmonize diagnosis and treatment, enhance the impartiality of clinical decisions, and enhance patient safety by reducing errors.(Davenport and Kalakota, 2019).AI can reduce the burden of administrative work done in clinical practice, thus allowing more time and resources for patient-centered initiatives and expanding affordable care options.(Khalifa et al., 2024)

AI-focused courses are necessary to keep up with AI's rapid development and ensure that graduates are well prepared to utilize it in an "ethical and responsible manner".(Kim et al., 2023)

As a high-performance assistant tool, are AI-based systems likely to replace orthodontists in specific tasks? With the rapid progression of AI technologies, the world evolves every day. Each day is different from yesterday, and there is so much room for improvement for tomorrow. Numerous studies have assessed the perspectives of dental experts and students regarding artificial intelligence technology. However, studies focusing on AI applications in orthodontics within the "Middle East and North Africa region" are limited, resulting in insufficient comprehensive data on this subject. To the best of our information, this research constitutes the first original study to be carried out in Iraq exploring the perception and attitudes toward implementing dental artificial intelligence among orthodontic specialists.

Aims and objectives

- **The aims of the study**

1) Inspecting the related perceptions and attitudes of Iraqi orthodontists (specialist academicians and clinicians with a higher education degree) toward using dental artificial intelligence in their clinical practice.
2) Highlighting specialist opinions toward AI-based applications and investigating their predictions regarding AI's future evolution in orthodontic practice to provide recommendations for improvements to existing AI applications.
3) Exploring potential avenues for interdisciplinary AI research opportunities in orthodontics.

- **Objectives**

1) Developing a validated survey study to investigate specialist orthodontists' knowledge and attitudes towards implementing AI-powered tools in orthodontic practice.
2) Content validation was conducted through a rigorous two-round process using Lawshe's method with the involvement of six orthodontic experts.
3) Face validity was evaluated using the percent agreement and Cohen's kappa statistics to assess inter-rater reliability, with two orthodontic experts involved in this evaluation.

LITERATURE REVIEW

1.1 Innovations in orthodontic assessment

1.1.1 The stated objectives of orthodontic assessment

In contemporary orthodontics, gathering diagnostic information to evaluate the craniofacial complex presents challenges. The cranial structures are intricately coordinated, performing numerous essential tasks and demonstrating dynamic interactions. Multiple neuromuscular activities regulate breathing, mastication, swallowing, speech, and facial expressions, and they must remain in equilibrium.(Lestrel, 1989)

Digital technology and three-dimensional (3D) imaging advancements have significantly enhanced the ability to combine dental documentation in various forms, leading to more precise assessment and analysis procedures.(Kau et al., 2011)

A significant amount of data is collected through an orthodontic clinical assessment, a review of two-dimensional radiographs, study models, and other essential patient records. Orthodontic recordings are often obtained in a static condition. Consequently, these data only partially represent craniofacial and dentoalveolar anatomy complexities, thereby constraining their diagnostic efficacy.(Broadbent, 1931; Mehta, 1993; Abdelkarim and Jerrold, 2017)

Capturing a 3-dimensional structure on a two-dimensional radiograph results in substantial data loss. A traditional two-dimensional radiograph is a " shadow" of a three-dimensional object, offering just minor or insufficient information about the projected structures. Consequently, specialists must regularly use their extensive knowledge and skills to "interpret" radiographs.(Han et al., 1991; DiFranco et al., 2001)

The conventional diagnostic approaches' ineffectiveness in accurately reflecting malocclusion and its related cranial features in all three planes may lead to an inadequate assessment or a misinterpretation.(McNamara , 2000; Lee et al., 2015a)

The conventional diagnostic approach enables orthodontists to evaluate malocclusions in a "feeding forward" manner, primarily based on the physician's perspective about the treatment and the orthodontist's level of expertise. Different opinions have largely emerged from this method, which frequently doesn't have an empirical foundation and favor mechanism-based over integrative treatment techniques.(Retrouvey and Abdallah, 2021) (Figure 1.1).

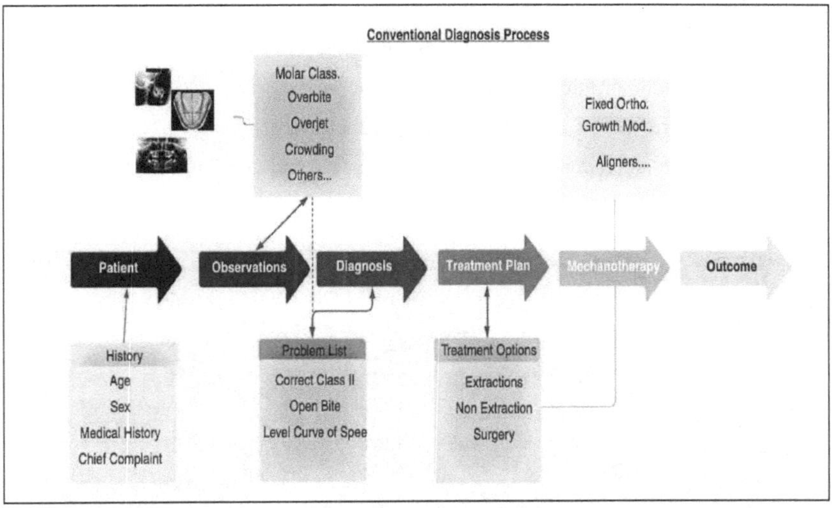

Figure 1.1: Evaluation and treatment planning in orthodontics follow traditional procedures. The patient is the starting point, and the outcome is the finishing touch of the process. This is a forward procedure implementing the "feeding forward" mechanism. No feedback approach is available.(Retrouvey et al., 2021a)

By integrating intraoral scan and cone beam computed tomography, orthodontists' diagnostic abilities have been greatly improved through three-dimensional assessment. Modern inventions enable the incorporation of substantial clinical information acquisitions, which facilitate numerous orthodontic simulations, modify treatment procedures, and perform in-house 3D printing (Hou et al., 2020; Retrouvey et al., 2021a).

The purposes of collecting and analyzing digital orthodontic records are as follows. (Retrouvey et al., 2021a) :

1. Archiving records securely.

2. In order to fully capture the specific cranial features and occlusion of every individual.
3. Exploring various treatment scenarios.
4. To formulate an extensive treatment program
5. Correlating the outcomes with different categories of malocclusions.
6. To enable an evaluation for treatment advancement.
7. Planning for orthognathic procedures.
8. To manufacture personalized and custom appliances.
9. To maintain collaboration with other fields of specialization. (Figures 1.2 and 1.3)

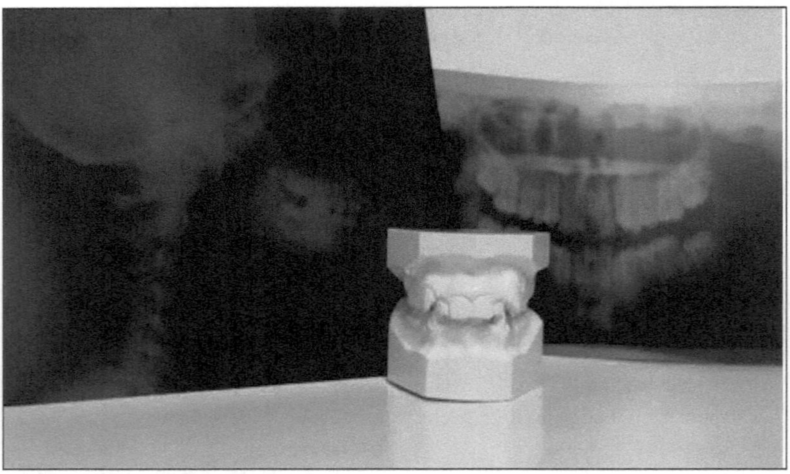

Figure 1.2: A compilation of diagnostic records, including a dental cast, cephalometric, and panoramic radiographs.(Retrouvey et al., 2021a)

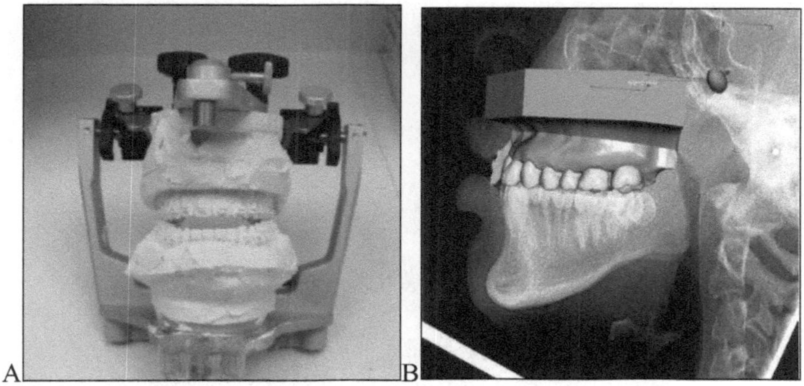

Figure 1.3: (A) A semi-adjustable articulator, while (B) a virtual three-dimensional articulator enables more precise spatial positioning of dental casts.(Retrouvey et al., 2021a)

1.1.2 The evolutionary process in orthodontic documentation over time

1.1.2.1 Assessment sheet

Data collection from patients has traditionally relied heavily on documentary assessment sheets. They comprise records of extraoral and intraoral examinations, a short questionnaire, medical history, and the patient's principal concerns. The obtained data are infrequently evaluated during treatment and seldom integrated into any database.(Retrouvey et al., 2021a)

1.1.2.2 Extra and intra-oral photograph

Dental photos were first used a few decades ago.(Terry et al., 2008), while extraoral images offer significant information about a patient's facial characteristics, intraoral images document the state and placement of teeth relative to one another and adjacent soft tissues.(Claman et al., 1990).Without precise calibration, dental photos do not provide quantifiable data. The data they provide is mainly qualitative, assisting clinicians in confirming their clinical evaluations of patients.(Bengel, 2000).(Figure 1.4)

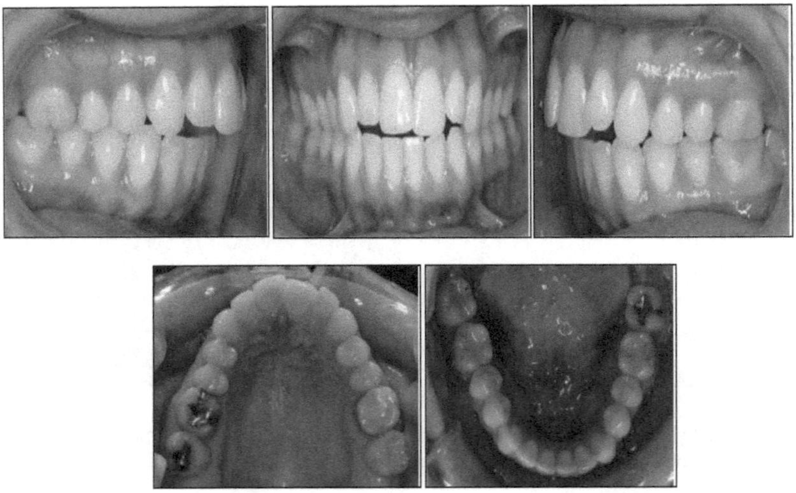

Figure 1.4: Intra-oral digital images. (Bengel, 2000)

1.1.2.3 Orthopantomogram (OPG) radiograph

A panoramic radiograph has multiple benefits for regular diagnostics, such as affordability and accessibility. It releases a small amount of radiation. Although it is regarded primarily as a diagnostic radiograph, it does not facilitate accurate and predictable assessments. Regardless of its advantages, the radiograph offers an inadequate visualization of the patient's anatomy or pathological conditions. Both erroneous positive and negative interpretations occur frequently. (Maestre-Ferrín et al., 2011)

For instance, the subsequent panoramic radiograph (Figure 1.5) illustrates unerupted maxillary canines but lacks spatial data regarding their relationship to the surrounding dentition. Assessing the condition of lateral incisor roots is notably difficult. Using CBCT enables orthodontists to evaluate their status precisely (Figure 1.6).(Tsolakis et al., 2018)

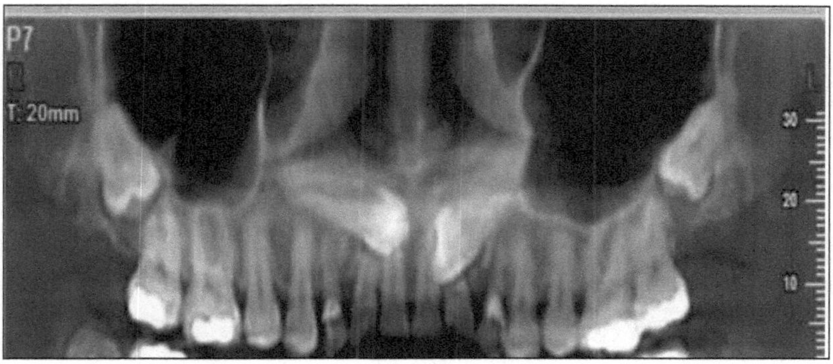

Figure 1.5: OPG showing up unerupted maxillary canines.(Tsolakis et al., 2018)

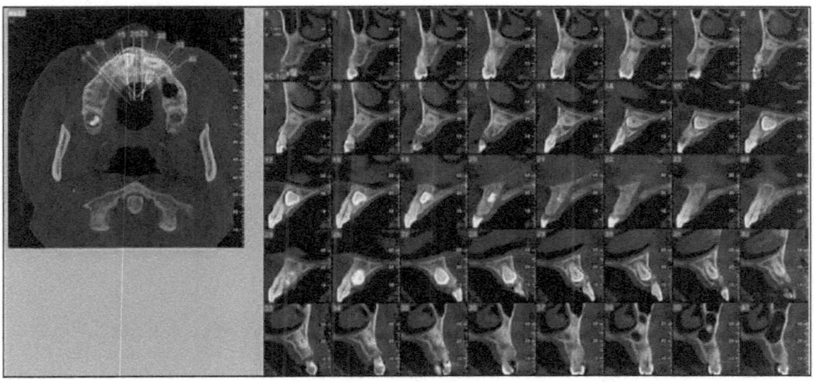

Figure 1.6: CBCT of the same patient shows resorption of the lateral incisor root.(Tsolakis et al., 2018)

1.1.2.4 Cephalometric X-ray

The lateral cephalometric x-ray illustrates an image of the whole craniofacial elements onto a sagittal two-dimensional axis.(Vandenberghe et al., 2010).It is primarily used for cephalometric evaluations to compare the patient's measurements with standard norms.(Steiner, 1953) (Figure 1.7).

Cephalograms are essential in orthodontic diagnosis because they allow for precise evaluation of the maxillary and mandibular arches with dental elements in vertical and anteroposterior directions.(Scheideman et al., 1980).While components that aren't positioned on the mid sagittal direction of the cranium are challenging to recognize, such as condyles, temporal fossa, and auditory meatus.(Ludlow et al., 2009).

	Value	Norm	Std Dev
SNA (°)	78.7	81.0	3.0
SNB (°)	71.9	78.0	3.0
ANB (°)	6.8	3.0	2.0
Facial Angle (FH-NPo) (°)	85.5	88.0	4.0
Wits Appraisal [Glupker]	-3.2	2.0	2.0
MP - SN (°)	47.3	33.0	3.0
Y-Axis (SGn-SN) (°)	75.6	60.0	4.0
U1 - NA (°)	23.2	23.0	6.0
L1 - NB (°)	32.4	27.5	5.0
Interincisal Angle (U1-L1	117.6	130.0	7.0
IMPA (L1-MP) (°)	693.3	91.4	4.0
Mandibular length (Co-G	109.8	122.3	4.0
Maxillary length (Co-A)	79.3	90.0	5.0

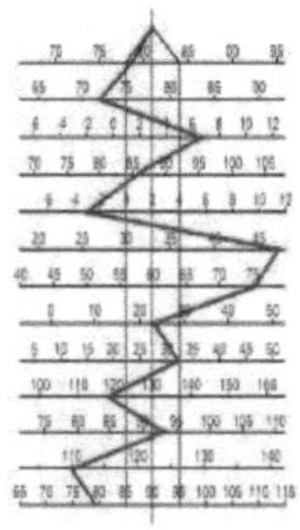

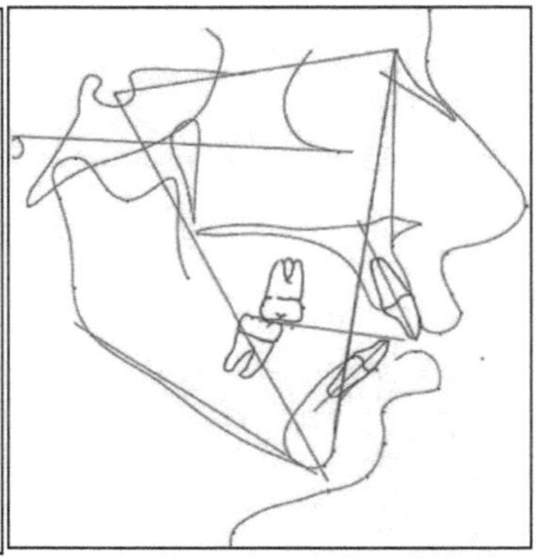

Figure 1.7: Tracing of cephalometric x-ray with a cephalometric analysis.(Steiner, 1953)

1.1.2.5 Orthodontic Diagnostic Models

They are beneficial for gaining information regarding the relative relationships of the dentition and facilitating its assessment with dentoalveolar components. Nonetheless, it is unfeasible to ascertain precise root locations and their relationships to adjacent dentoalveolar structures utilizing orthodontic study models. Conducting an orthodontic treatment plan simulation on plaster models is exceedingly difficult. Generally, they possess lower diagnostic qualifications relative to their digital equivalents. (Ackerman, 2003) (Figure 1.8)

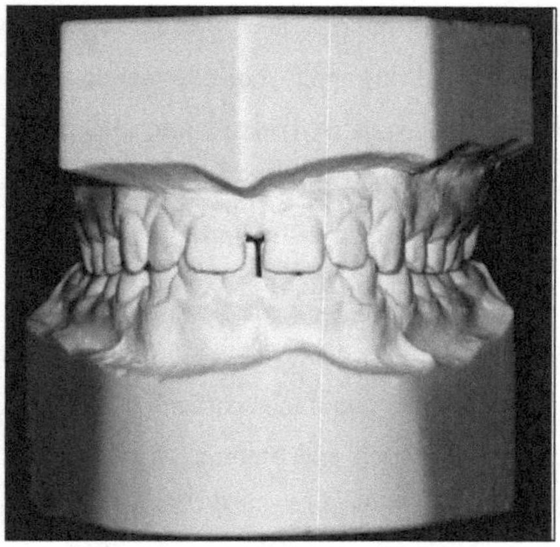

Figure 1.8: Diagnostic cast trimmed according to orthodontic criteria. No relationship is present to the surrounding cranial structures.(Ackerman, 2003)

In summary, the traditional diagnostic process had previously enabled clinicians to achieve reasonably accurate diagnoses. However, its reliability has faced some challenges in the contemporary digital world. Even with a meticulously performed clinical evaluation, standard orthodontic records do not substantially enhance diagnostic capability.(Beglin et al., 2001).This may be attributed to a substantial loss of clinical information from these documentation formats.(Dolce et al., 2012)

1.1.3 The foundation of a three-dimensional digital orthodontic document: a superior approach to assess the craniofacial structure

Digital technology is characterized by precision, quickness, and consistency.(Paredes et al., 2006).A digital assessment form, intraoral photos, oral scans "in STL file format" and 3D radiographs such as "CBCT in DICOM format" could be combined into a unified document for the assessment phase of the orthodontic procedures using practice management software.(Xiao et al., 2020). Subsequently, the data set is imported into "Computer-Aided Design, CAD software" to generate a personalized and animated three-dimensional representation of the patient. The potential to examine various elements of dental occlusion is the most promising application of computerized data because this would allow the physician to create a personalized orthodontic strategy for each patient, enabling simultaneous three-dimensional evaluations of craniofacial features, occlusion, and dentoalveolar measurement to propose the most suitable approach and alternative possibilities.(Yagi et al., 2010; Takada, 2016)

Combining DICOM and STL files enables orthodontists to correlate clinical dentition crowns and roots with adjacent craniofacial structures. Given that the software can continuously document the direction and amount of each orthodontic movement, the subsequent logical step is to view this aggregated data into predictive models to enhance our understanding of potential relationships between all diagnostic elements and the resultant orthodontic movements.(Kunz et al., 2020).(Figure 1.9).

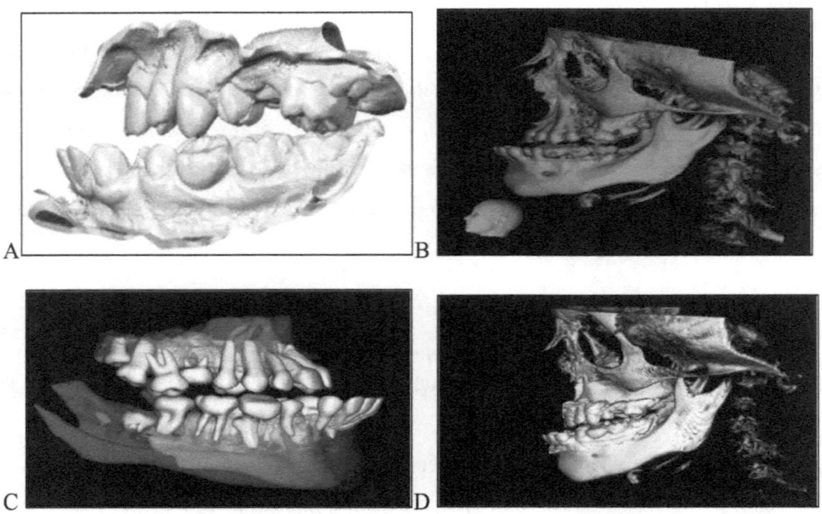

Figure 1.9: (A) STL files generated by intraoral scanning. (B) Patient's cone beam CT scan. (C) The density tool is used to segment the dentition in cone beam computed tomography. The teeth's position in three-dimensional space is easily observed. (D)Integrating STL data and DICOM file.(Kunz et al., 2020)

This can allow orthodontists to relate diagnostic data with treatment outcomes precisely. These observations will assist in more effectively identifying patterns that may have been previously missed using traditional two-dimensional diagnostic procedures, where most diagnostic assessments are unidirectional and based on the personal experiences of orthodontists, with outcomes of treatment not utilized as feedback strategies to enhance the upcoming outcomes.(Zhao et al., 2017). (Figure 1.10) outlines the outcome loops that can be used as feedback to enhance the orthodontist's diagnosis and treatment plan and to support communication with the patient.

Furthermore, treatment progress can be consistently monitored using sequential intraoral scans, while patient files remain instantly accessible chairside for reference and reviewing.(Retrouvey et al., 2021b)

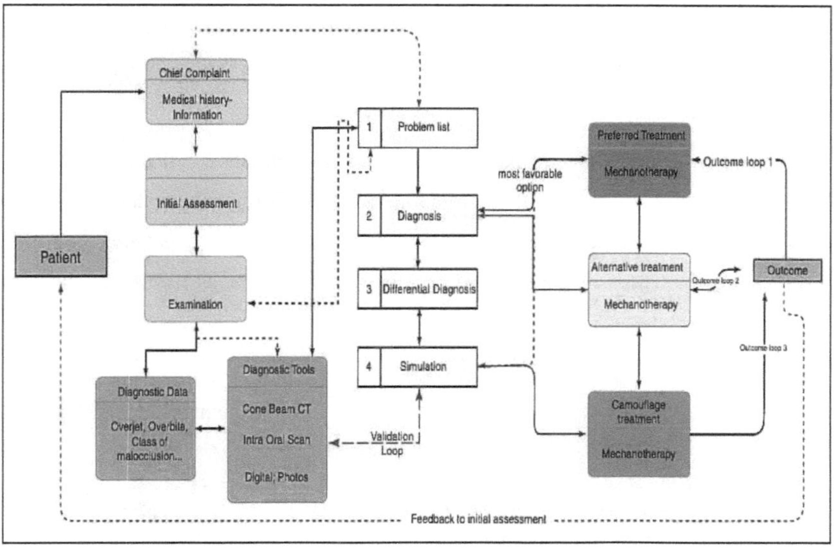

Figure 1.10: Three-dimensional diagnostic procedure with a feedback mechanism enabling the experts to evaluate and ascertain the efficacy of the treatment strategy.(Zhao et al., 2017)

1.2 Revolution of orthodontic assessment in the era of artificial intelligence technology

1.2.1 What are intelligent systems?

The next evolution in digital diagnosis is the implementation of artificial intelligence. Dave Waters remarked, "Predicting the future is not magic; it is artificial intelligence". Artificial intelligence represents a branch of software engineering centred on developing intelligent systems with human-like cognitive abilities and actions. AI can analyze intricate medical data; it has the potential to reveal valuable connections within datasets, which could potentially be employed for the course of treatment, dental evaluation along with the prediction of the results across diverse clinical scenarios. AI includes applications like understanding language, the educational process, and figuring out solutions. While intelligent technology is shown by the robots, human intelligence is displayed by humans. Essentially, AI relies on "computer-trained algorithms" that imitate human intelligence.(Ramesh et al., 2004; Jaju, et al., 2023)

Algorithms, which are "sets of instructions", power the artificial intelligence system by directing a computer's behavior. Key algorithms used in artificial intelligence include decision trees for decision-making, neural networks for identifying patterns, and deep learning algorithms for complex procedures like speech and image detection.(Orhan and Jagtap, 2023).(Figure 1.11)

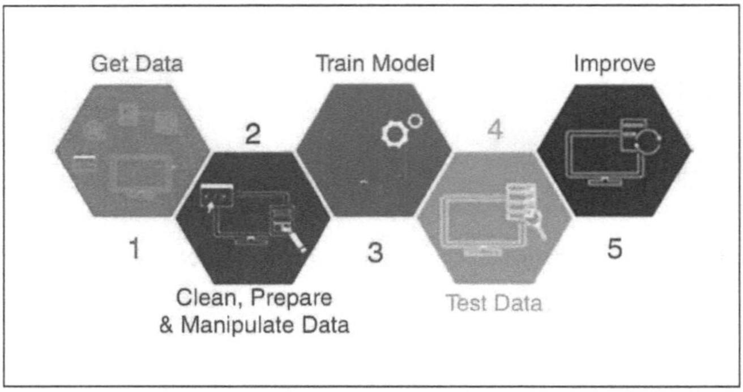

Figure 1.11: A diagram showing the phases involved in artificial intelligence software creation. (Jaju, et al., 2023)

With AI, orthodontists can explore different treatment possibilities, incorporating feedback from the results to develop more sophisticated and Advanced learning models.(Martina et al., 2006).(Figure 1.12)

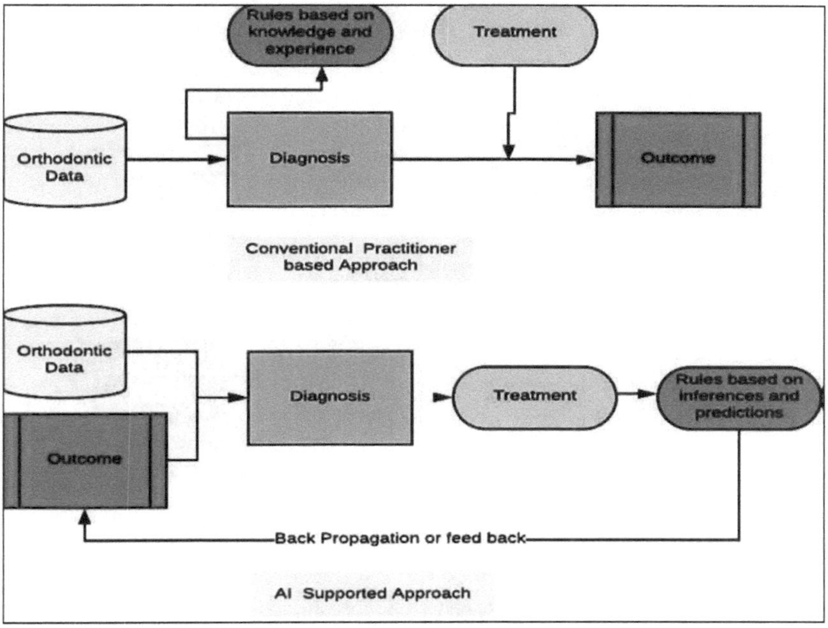

Figure 1.12: Conventional-based approach versus artificial intelligence-driven approach for evaluation and treatment strategy in orthodontics.(Wei et al., 2020)

1.2.2 How does artificial intelligence work?

Through the analysis of extensive information sets, intelligent machines are capable of being programmed for offering more reliable and precise outcomes for orthodontic diagnoses and treatment plans. It employs neural networks and deep learning in order to forecast a suitable approach for each particular occlusion scenario. It organizes multiple categories of data processing, considering factors like crowding, overbite, and overjet while assigning a weight to each variable.(Kulikowski, 1980; Jaju, et al., 2023)

Progress in this area will come from feeding extensive clinical information within the artificial neural network models, allowing them for accurately calculating the likelihood concerning the positive results depending upon the effective management of a wide range of improper alignment.(Retrouvey et al., 2021a).(Figure 1.13)

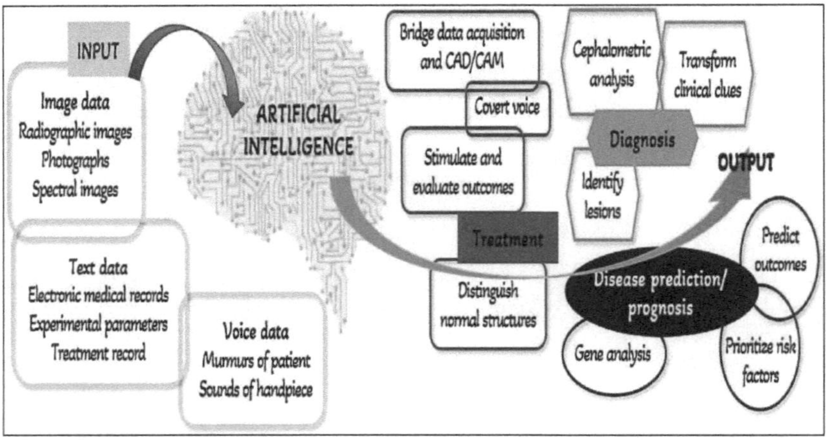

Figure 1.13: Artificial intelligence operates like machines and is structured around three core stages: input, processing, and output. (Agrawal and Nikhade, 2022)

There are several types of AI, including: -

1) Machine learning (ML) constitutes a subset portion of artificial intelligence, which concentrates upon the development of machines with algorithms which automatically improve their performance through entered information instead of relying on manually coded algorithms.ML is widely applied in “image recognition, natural language processing, and predictive analytics.” Such as integrating intelligent ML and extensive cone beam computed tomography examination information may improve the prediction of face development, with facilitating an additional precise management strategy.

Unlike what some may assume, machine learning relies on extensive data input and can only identify structured, semi-repetitive patterns independently. It does not possess "true perception or intuition." Therefore, an orthodontist's knowledge and experience are vital components in machine learning development.

2) Deep learning (DL) is a particular category of ML and another form of representation learning which relies on "artificial neural networks", that mimic the functioning of the cognitive system of the human being. DL algorithms enhance their capabilities by processing enormous quantities of materials and information, making it possible for carrying out sophisticated functions.(W. J. Park & Park, 2018; Faber et al., 2019; Ko et al., 2019; Schwendicke et al., 2020; Hung et al., 2020; Khanagar et al., 2021b; Shan et al., 2021; Carrillo-Perez et al., 2022).In healthcare imaging, deep learning algorithms primarily use CNNs, or the "convolutional neural networks," for obtaining increased diagnostic accuracy.(Rajpurkar et al., 2018; Yu et al., 2022).(Figures 1.14 and 1.15)

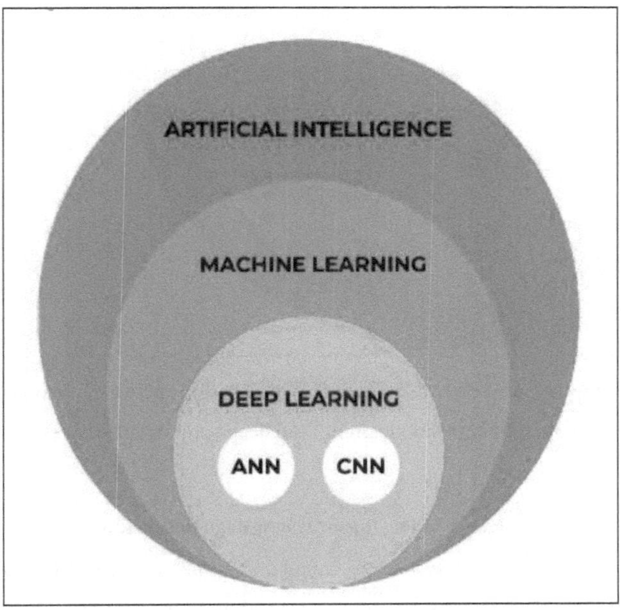

Figure 1.14: Optimized artificial intelligence representation.(Kazimierczak et al., 2024)

3) Representation learning is a type of "machine learning" that does not require a data preparation procedure. In this approach, the model independently sorts the input data according to its features. When sufficient training examples are available, a representation learning-based system can yield superior classification results compared to one relying on manual data manipulation or transformation. (Akkaya et al., 2023).(Figure 1.15)

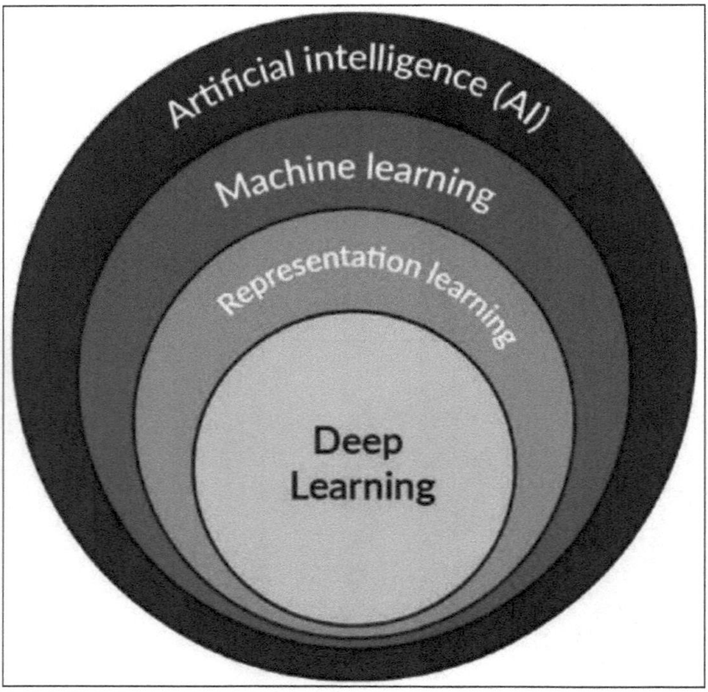

Figure 1.15: A graphic diagram demonstrates the "relationship between artificial intelligence, machine learning, representation learning, and deep learning". (Akkaya et al., 2023)

4) Another field of artificial intelligence is the "**natural language processing,**" which is particularly concentrated on facilitating systems to comprehend and analyze words used by humans. AI-powered machines that are providing technical assistance rely heavily on

natural language processing systems to automate jobs like interpreting languages, word categorization, and identification of speech. (Orhan and Jagtap, 2023)

5) Robotics is one of the most prominent fields of AI. It involves programming machines to carry out activities that typically require human expertise and intelligence. These robots are programmed to handle operations in fields such as production and transportation, helping automate repetitive functions and increase operational efficiency.(Orhan and Jagtap, 2023)

Artificial intelligence has evolved in three distinct stages. The first generation, which emerged in the 1980s and 1990s, relied on predetermined regulations to analyze the information and formulate the results. The next phase, in the two-thousands, implemented the "concept of learning," which means that computers can independently create outcomes according to predetermined guidelines derived from information input by humans. Presently, we are living in the era of the third generation, which is all about "deep learning." With DL, algorithms can comprehend different instructions, evaluate distinctive information, and produce outcomes without ever needing human intervention.(Jaju, et al., 2023)

1.3 AI and its applications in orthodontics

Artificial intelligence has a significant impact on orthodontic education and practice. Integrating AI in orthodontics signifies a significant transformation, optimizing workflows, increasing accuracy, and ultimately elevating the efficacy of orthodontic treatment. The connection between orthodontics and AI is progressing with continual technological improvements to transform the dental healthcare field, providing patients with more customized and effective solutions. (Alowais et al., 2023; Liu et al., 2023)

Most areas of intelligent system usage in orthodontics may generally be categorized into four primary areas: examination and planning of the treatment procedures, assessment of the anticipated outcomes, treatment follow-up, patient motivation, and communication.(Bichu et al., 2025).(Figure 1.16). (Figure 1.17) Presents a diagram summarizing different scenarios of intelligent system use in orthodontic practice.

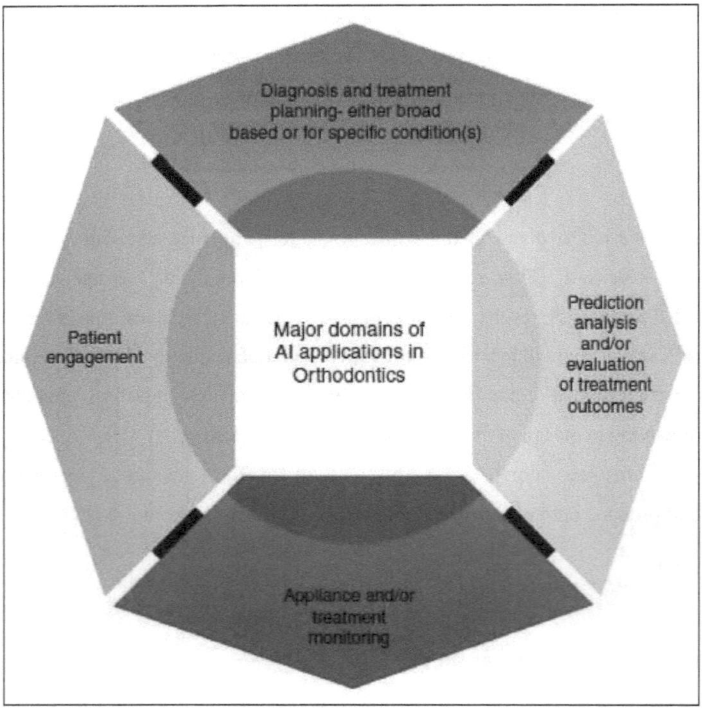

Figure 1.16: Key areas of intelligence system implementation in clinical practice.(Bichu et al., 2025)

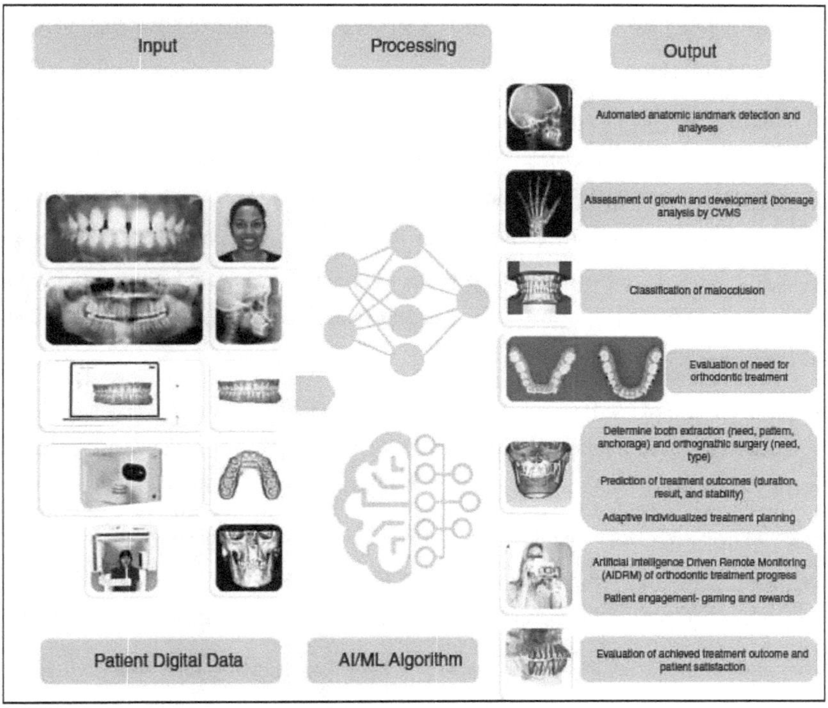

Figure 1.17: Different domains of intelligent system utilization in orthodontics practice.(Bichu et al., 2025)

In orthodontics, the following are the predominant applications of artificial intelligence technology:

1.3.1 Automatic lateral cephalometric digitization, tracing, and analysis

Cephalometric tracing relied solely on traditional tracing and landmark detection for many years; however, the advancement of artificial intelligence technology has made this a viable alternative.(Schwendicke et al., 2019; Monill-González et al., 2021; Subramanian et al., 2022). Recent developments in computer technology enable gathering digital and /or scanned lateral cephalometric images within database servers, facilitating automated landmark detection and cephalometric assessment, including tracing and accurate measurements. (Kunz et al., 2020)

A variety of web-based software and apps have been developed with similar objectives, including "CephX (ORCA dental AI, Las Vegas, NV), WebCeph and AutoCAD software, Dolphin Imaging, Dentofacial Planner, Quick Ceph, and FACAD, AudaxCeph, OrisCeph Rx". (Meriç and Naoumova, 2020; Yu et al., 2020; Juneja et al., 2021; Yassir et al., 2022).Reviews of these software applications show significant potential in enhancing and optimizing Professional orthodontic practices.(Nishimoto et al., 2019; Park et al., 2019)(Figure 1.18)

Numerous research studies have evaluated the utility of artificial intelligence in landmark placement. After examining "400–500" lateral cephalometric x-rays, they demonstrated a promising accuracy range of "88.43% to 92%". (Kim et al., 2020; Lee et al., 2020a)

Even while conventional identification is still likely the most prevalent approach, the shift to artificial Intelligence-assisted analysis offers benefits that make it less time-consuming and reduce both accidental and methodical individual errors.(Subramanian et al., 2022)

Although artificial intelligence using ML and DL has shown remarkable accuracy in calculating cephalometric results, orthodontic specialists still need to verify the location of every landmark following the automated identification process. (Arik et al., 2017; Subramanian et al., 2022)

After evaluating Convolutional neural network-related systems, Yu and colleagues found that the vertical and anteroposterior skeletal assessment resolution, specificity, and accuracy were higher than (90%). (Yu et al., 2020)

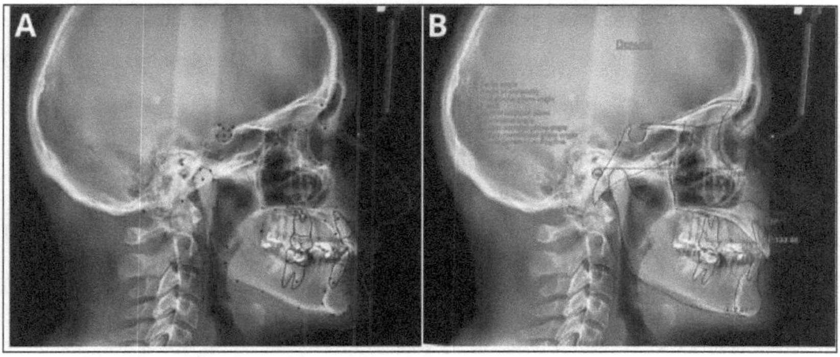

Figure 1.18: Automated lateral cephalometric tracing and analysis conducted with (A) CephX and (B) WebCeph for 18 years old male. Red-coloured assessments of the Downs analysis outcomes are those that fall outside the typical range.(Kazimierczak et al., 2024)

1.3.2 Orthopantomogram (OPG) Radiograph

O.P.G images present a significant challenge for analysis due to the vast amount of data they contain, which encompasses dental and skeletal diseases, variations, deviations, and periodontal conditions or for the inevitable overlap of different structures in the anatomy that may affect the overall quality of the images.(Hwang et al., 2017; Schwendicke et al., 2019). In such a situation, Artificial intelligence could significantly aid dental physicians by supporting rather than substituting human input.(Chandrashekar et al., 2022)

Artificial intelligence can be utilized in the following areas. (Hwang et al., 2017; Schwendicke et al., 2019; Lee et al., 2020b) :

1) Segmentation of the specific items, focusing on the precise shape of anatomy or abnormal conditions.
2) The categorization of these particular items.
3) Identifying specific anatomical structures such as teeth and condyles.
4) Detecting abnormalities, including decreased bone density, fractures in the bone, apical infection, and cavities.
5) Consideration of the forensic objective.

Since detecting abnormalities presents greater challenges and likely necessitates additional expertise to enhance final results, DL has primarily been utilized in examinations for dental assessment, as indicated in existing studies. (Krois et al., 2019)

Given the encouraging outcomes of tooth segmentation reliability (87%) and the competence in dental recognition (96.94%), it is predicted that all AI technologies would facilitate orthodontic procedures in practical settings. (Krois et al., 2021; Hou et al., 2023)

1.3.3 Cone beam computed tomography (CBCT)

The utilization of three-dimensional evaluations of CBCT within the field of Orthodontics has notably been increased with the implementation of AI techniques. Cone beam computed tomography imaging analysis presents a greater level of complexity and requires more time for a thorough examination compared to traditional two-dimensional X-rays. The implementation of Artificial Intelligence-based tools has streamlined this process. The automated segmentation of craniofacial structures using artificial intelligence (AI) techniques has shown significant progress, exhibiting improved time efficiency and a greater degree of precision. This will assist researchers and orthodontists in navigating this complicated and demanding job.(Miranda et al., 2023a) (Figure 1.19)

Apical pathology is detected in CBCT imaging with 92.8 % precision. The study by (Orhan et al., 2020) , indicated that AI approaches exhibited not any statistically significant variance in measurement results when compared to traditional techniques.

The comprehensive diagnostic efficiency involving both groups—one with artificial intelligence (AI) assistance and the other without- was examined in an oral cone-beam computed tomography evaluation in an article published by (Ezhov et al., 2021).The research's artificial intelligence (AI) program comprised applications for verifying apical lesions, periodontal disease, cavities, teeth identification and measurement, and dental and facial segmentation. The findings indicated that AI technology markedly enhanced the examination abilities of dental professionals, demonstrating superior diagnostic accuracy values in the artificial Intelligence-based group compared to the unassisted group.

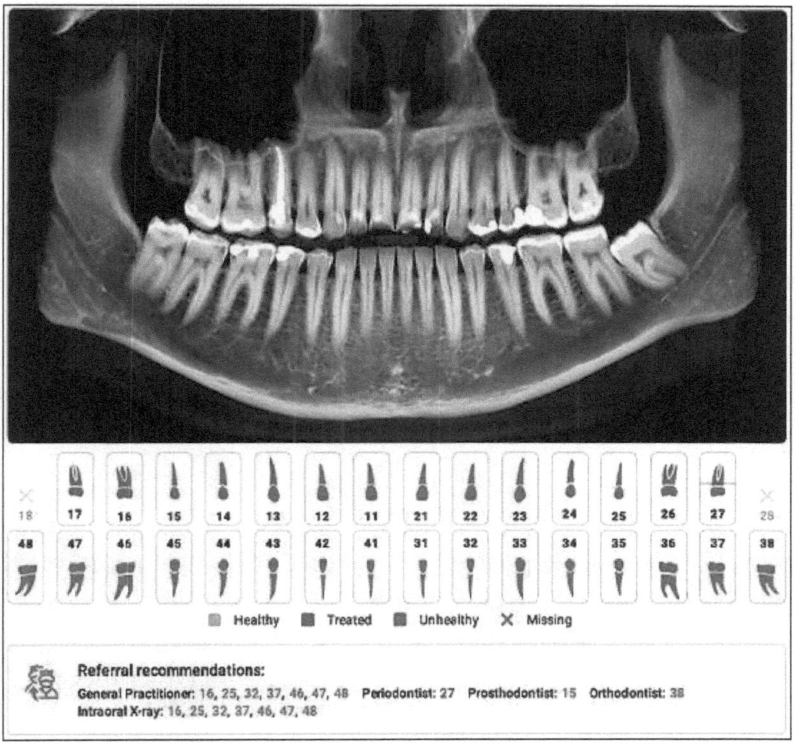

Figure 1.19: An automated assessment submitted reports concerning "CBCT scan" obtained before the procedures of orthodontic treatment for a "24-year-old male". The program efficiently detected absent tooth No.18 with tooth No.28, along with alterations in the rest of the teeth, which mainly included restorations and attritions. The software program has advised extra assessments as needed. (Kazimierczak et al., 2024)

1.3.4 Implementation of AI for virtual surgical planning and estimating the attractiveness of the face following orthognathic surgery

The incorporation of AI has brought about a paradigm shift in orthodontic surgery, which is a complicated area of orthodontics that includes surgically fixing abnormalities in the jaws. Artificial intelligence can identify essential structures, facilitating the anticipation of the need for surgical treatment.(Wong et al., 2023)

Furthermore, providing artificial intelligence with photographs of faces can produce precise findings and make it easier to identify the profile that might benefit from orthognathic procedures.(Lee et al., 2020c)

Virtual surgical planning employs intelligent system algorithms for the simulation of operations and the prediction of results.(Tahir et al., 2024).Surgeons can benefit from the use of structural three-dimensional (virtual reconstruction from CBCT) since it enables the three-dimensional assessment of patients' maxillofacial characteristics, enhancing identification and analysis of the effects of treatment. (Wang et al., 2021) has employed the DL-powered auto-segmentation modality of CBCT to examine the maxillary forms in all their dimensions, asymmetry, and abnormalities in unilateral cleft palate (UCP), and considerable hypoplasia was detected in the region of the cleft.

In another research, an investigation has been designed to create an AI automatic diagnostic model to detect Adenoid hypertrophy (AH) utilizing lateral cephalometric X-rays. Implementing artificial intelligence (AI) in the screening of Adenoid hypertrophy can facilitate a more rapid diagnosis in children, thereby minimizing the significant effects of mouth breathing and obstructive sleep apnea on their facial and bodily development. (Nauwelaers et al., 2021; Zhao et al., 2021)

A research project employed an ANN-powered algorithm to anticipate images of post-surgical treatment. The predicted images showed positive outcomes with an accuracy rate of above (80%). (Lu et al., 2009). These findings were comparable to another artificial intelligence study by (Patcas et al., 2019) that described how orthognathic procedures affected the face. (Figure 1.20) illustrates AI integration for orthognathic surgery procedures.

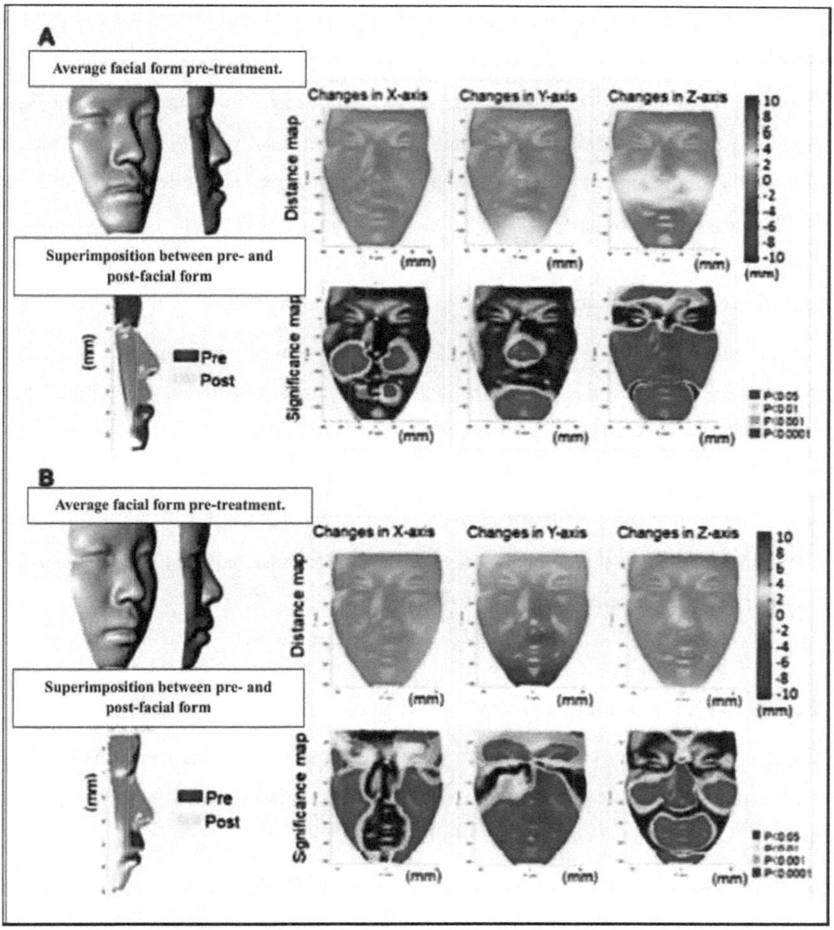

Figure 1.20: Implementation of artificial intelligence for preparing orthognathic surgery and estimating facial alterations for cases with Facio-skeletal malformation, including "pre-treatment, superimposition, and post-treatment ".(Rokaya et al., 2024)

1.3.5 Estimating the demand for orthodontic intervention and formulating clinical decisions

To assist orthodontists in making decisions, AI-powered tools have recently been employed as a (clinical decision support system). The most recent innovations aim to address the limitations of inaccurate indices. A research project implementing artificial intelligence (AI) techniques was developed to estimate the necessity for orthodontic interventions. The system has shown effectiveness and yielded excellent outcomes.(Thanathornwong, 2018)

An artificial neural network-driven system for orthodontics was employed in another investigation; the outcomes proved the model's exceptional effectiveness and high levels of precision for assessing both anchoring modalities in addition to extraction and non-extraction patterns. (Li et al., 2019)

According to the research findings, these models can be helpful tools for providing alternative supplemental judgments for beginner orthodontists in determining the necessity for orthodontic treatment.(Khanagar et al., 2021b)

1.3.6 Decision for extraction versus non-extraction treatment approach

Choosing the best course of action for a patient in many debatable situations can be a challenging task. Academic education and expertise can influence the type of treatment modality that orthodontists favor. (Etemad et al., 2021)

An ANN has been employed to determine the necessity of extracting teeth using diagnostic characteristics and lateral cephalometric analysis. It has demonstrated 80% accuracy in identifying the best course of action for 200 cases with different scenarios, ages ranging from 11 to 15.(Xie et al., 2010)

In South Korea, another research recruited 156 cases with twelve lateral cephalometric x-rays and six other medical characteristics to predict the possibility of treating the case, whether with or without extraction, using an ANN algorithm. 93% of the time, the algorithm correctly identified the most suitable course of action for the relevant patient.(Shafi et al., 2024)

1.3.7 Estimating the extent of cervical vertebrae maturation (CVM)

Since age in years has not been shown to be a good indicator of growth stages, determining the cervical vertebrae maturation is crucial. (Alkhal et al., 2008).Nowadays, the most accurate way to assess a person's physiological development is to study variations in and maturity phases of the vertebrae in the cervical region. (Litsas and Ari-Demirkaya, 2010; Navlani and Makhija, 2013)

It has been found that artificial neural network-driven algorithms showed an average success rate of 77.02% in estimating CVM.(Kök et al., 2019). (Figure 1.21). These findings are comparable to those of similar research in which the result was even better.(Makaremi et al., 2019)

In conclusion, artificial intelligence-powered models effectively identify CVMs and may benefit orthodontic professionals more.(Khanagar et al., 2021b)

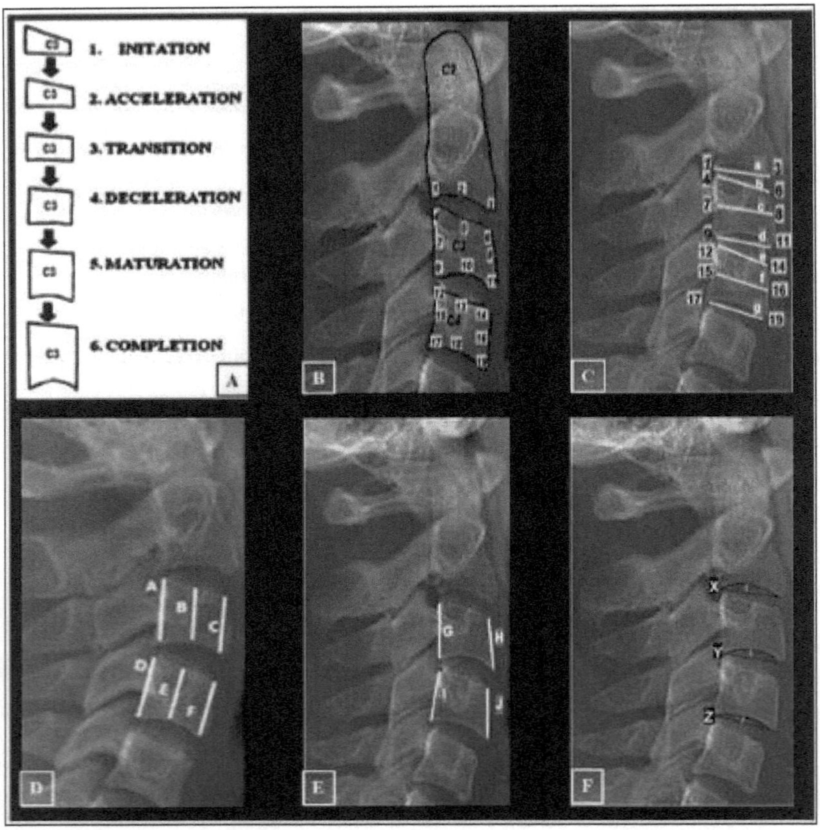

Figure 1.21: A graphic illustration showing the physical dimensions between various cervical vertebrae regions. (A) stages of cervical vertebrae maturation, (B) degree of curvature on the lower border of cervical vertebrae,(C and F) show evaluation on the horizontal axis (the spaces between cervical vertebrae), and (D and E) show the assessment on the vertical axis. (Kök et al., 2019)

1.3.8 Handling the situations of unerupted canines

Unerupted canines require a multidisciplinary technique for the best esthetic and gingival results. The duration of treatment depends on various factors, including the distance of the canine from the neighboring incisors.(Bahaa et al., 2011)

Different plane evaluations using O.P.G. and lateral cephalogram X-rays can support estimating the probability of unerupted canines' occurrence. By 83% precision and efficiency, random forests-based algorithms accurately predicted the canine's erupting situation.(Asiri et al., 2020)

An AI system based on ML, known as "Learning-based multi-source Integration framework for Segmentation," was integrated with the cone beam computed tomography to measure maxillary variability in asymmetrical canine eruption cases.(Chen et al., 2020)

1.3.9 Estimating dental dimension in developing occlusion

Estimating the space available for the unerupted permanent teeth is crucial for occlusal harmony and management in the mixed dentition period.

The most frequently utilized approaches for estimation are (Palanivel et al., 2021) :

A) Different analysis methods for developing occlusion

B) Periapical and panoramic x-rays

C) Using both of the methods mentioned above

(Moghimi et al., 2012) carried out research that quantified the dimensions of unerupted permanent canines and premolars. "ANN-hybrid system and genetic algorithms" were implemented. According to this research's findings, ANN is guaranteed to be a more accurate method than linear regression studies for estimating the sizes of unerupted canines with first and second premolars.

1.3.10 Selection of the Suitable Headgear Appliance

Headgear is an extraoral orthopedic appliance that can prevent forward growth of the maxilla and facilitate distalization and anchorage devices. It is available in high, medium, and low pull modalities. Junior orthodontists may find it challenging to select the most appropriate type. For supporting the clinical decisions in choosing the best headgear modality that suits the individual patient's requirements, a model powered by artificial intelligence was developed. The system's judgments were assessed by eight professional experts, confirming the AI system's efficiency and reliability.(Akçam and Takada, 2002)

1.3.11 Assessing the soft tissue profile response to orthodontic intervention

The harmonious and balanced configuration of facial soft tissues, including the association between the chin, nose, and upper and lower lips, is crucial for achieving optimal dental and facial aesthetics.(Palanivel et al., 2021)

ANNs have been validated as capable of estimating the future alterations in the contour of the lips after orthodontic interventions.(Nanda et al., 2015)

Another study implemented an ANNs for the purpose of evaluating the proportion of the face before and after surgical treatment by scores from zero to 100. The outcomes indicated that the recorded ratings demonstrated a substantial enhancement in the appearance of the face.(Patcas et al., 2019)

1.3.12 Estimating the appropriate force system in orthodontic treatment

A key component of orthodontics biomechanics is applying the proper force, which helps achieve the desired dental movement and alignment, appropriate soft tissue adaptation, and orthopedic improvement.(Palanivel et al., 2021)

An ANN-based AI system designed by (Kazem et al., 2010) for identifying a relevant optimal force of the "T-retraction Loop", it achieved favorable results and proved efficient.

1.3.13 Management of TMJ disorders

TMJ diseases, which affect between 5% to 12% of individuals, are considered among the 2nd predominant muscular and skeletal disorders. Temporomandibular joint osteoarthritis can be diagnosed by using automated deep ANN systems.(Lee et al., 2020d).(Figure 1.22)

An artificial intelligent system that includes information other than photographs, such as symptoms, clinical characteristics and manifestations, and individual patient characteristics and medical history, would significantly improve future diagnostic accuracy.(Shoukri et al., 2019). Artificial intelligence-driven photographs of the temporomandibular joint also offer insights into the medical signs of temporomandibular joint disorders and osteoarthritis, as well as their possible links to causative variables, including antibody reactions and gene mutations.(Khan et al., 2022)

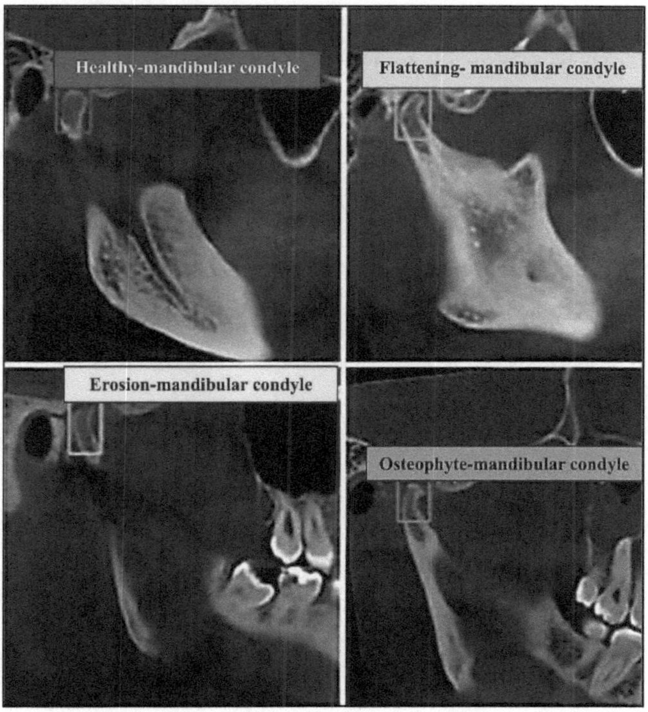

Figure 1.22: Temporomandibular joint osteoarthritis (TMJ-OA) can be effectively identified via CBCT photos using CranioCatch AI software. (Jagtap et al., 2023)

1.3.14 Individual patient monitoring

Fortunately, new developments in orthodontics, like clear aligners and self-ligating appliances, as well as telecommunications, have contributed to orthodontic patient monitoring. (Caruso et al., 2021)

Individual patient monitoring has advantages, including decreasing patient chairside time, increasing patient compliance, rapidly diagnosing orthodontic emergency situations, minimizing orthodontic instances of relapse, controlling the fitness of aligners, and enhancing dental health. (Kazimierczak et al., 2024)

1.3.15 Treatment with clear aligner system

AI-assisted orthodontic management has been popular for an extended duration. Several organizations manufacturing aligners use artificial intelligence techniques to enhance orthodontic design, thereby streamlining the process for orthodontic professionals.(Jorge et al., 2019)

Invisalign® is widely recognized as the leading aligner technique by implementing computerized simulated treatment planning and stereolithographic development. It has evolved into a broad name for numerous premium products utilizing computer-aided design innovation. (Lagravère and Flores-mir, 2005; Malik et al., 2013; Weir, 2017)

A software known as "The Clincheck® program, developed by Align Technology in Santa Clara, CA, USA", computes the necessary motion for every particular tooth, the fundamental mechanics involved in executing that motion, with the design and the technical specifications of the aligner. (Tamer et al., 2019).(Figure 1.23)

However, the AI algorithms powering these programs cannot replace professional orthodontists when formulating clinical decisions and planning treatment steps.(Fawaz et al., 2023)

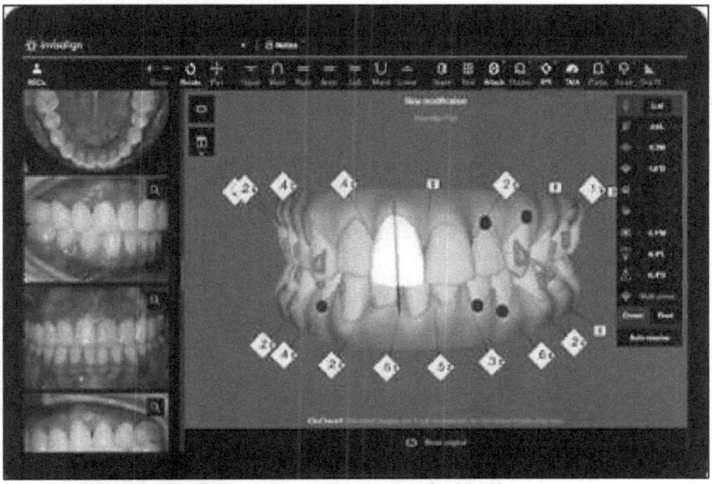

Figure 1.23: Clincheck® program. (Tamer et al., 2019)

1.3.16 Management of cleft lip and palate

The care and therapeutic management of people with lip and palate clefts abnormalities is being revolutionized by a smart AI approach. Advances in artificial intelligence can greatly enhance the complicated and diverse management protocols.(Tahir et al., 2024).(Figure 1.24)

A DL-based program had been created to define multiple defects of the cleft lip and palate by examining O.P.G x-rays for 383 individuals with alveolar clefts, including and not including palatal clefts, and 210 individuals with no cleft abnormality. Deep Learning software showed more precision and actually exceeded that of human observers.(Kuwada et al., 2021)

In a similar manner, innovative development in the assessment of asymmetrical cleft palate was achieved by utilizing deep learning techniques and cone beam computed tomography. This approach outperformed conventional techniques with an amazing overall segmentation and categorization performance of 96%.(Wang et al., 2021)

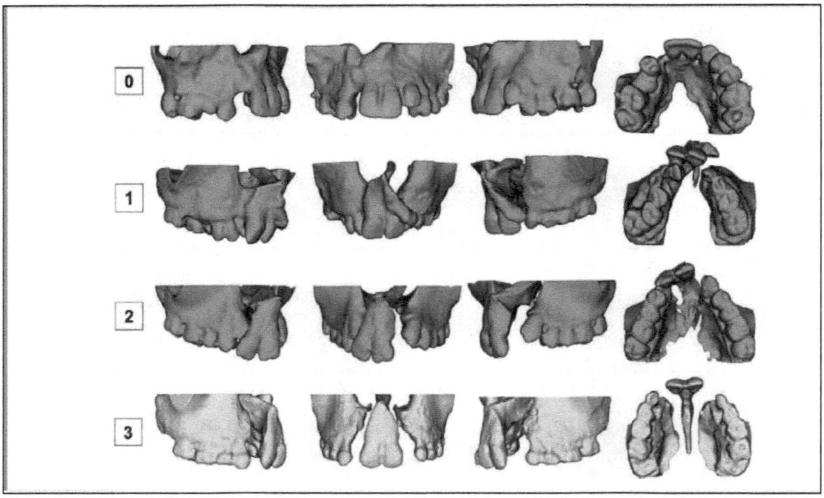

.Figure 1.24: Three-dimensional models were used to diagnose the seriousness of the cleft anomaly. The degree of severity was categorized on a scale from 0 to 3, with 0 representing a lower degree and 3 indicating a higher level of severity. (Miranda et al., 2023b)

1.3.17 Examination and management of the airway

The implementation of automatic airway investigation represents a noteworthy advancement of artificial intelligence in orthodontics, especially in evaluating and managing airway blockages. Conventional approaches for assessing the respiratory area, including lateral cephalometric examination and three-dimensional visualization, require significant time investment and are susceptible to subjective errors by individuals. ML-based software automatically diagnoses airway issues with good precision using three-dimensional scans and lateral cephalometric X-rays. (Tahir et al., 2024)

CNNs for automated airway investigation using cone-beam computed tomography displayed outstanding reliability, markedly decreasing the time needed for evaluation in contrast with traditional approaches. This progress facilitates the determination of obstructive sleep apnea (OSA) and the formulation of orthodontic procedures that consider airway functioning.(Tsolakis et al., 2022).(Figure 1.25)

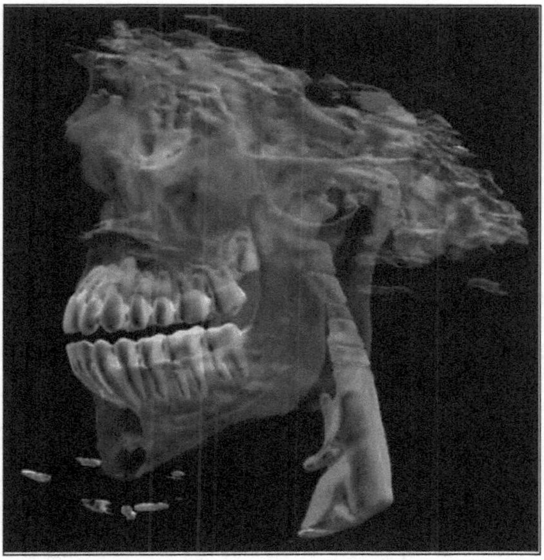

Figure 1.25: Three-dimensional airway evaluation utilizing CBCT through an artificial intelligence system. (Jaju, et al., 2023)

1.3.18 Analysis of the shape of the palate

The palate configuration is significant for orthodontic professionals, serving as a key area for examining and analyzing the results of treatment options such as expanding the maxilla. The anatomy of the palate is associated with the architecture of the face and is influenced by multiple variables, including dental occlusion and breathing habits.(Albalawi and Alamoud, 2022)

Palatal dimension, size, and height are typically incorporated in palatal evaluations. These evaluations frequently necessitate a higher level of expertise and are often prone to inspector mistakes. The latest technological developments have led to the creation of artificial intelligence tools tailored explicitly for palatal form assessment. For assessing the palatal form, DL-powered systems had been created. This design exhibited outstanding reliability along with excellent precision.(Croquet et al., 2021)

1.3.19 Retention in Orthodontics

Retainers are inactive items designed to maintain and preserve dental alignment after the intensive orthodontic treatment stage. Artificial intelligence can assist with evaluating retention, producing various kinds of retainer designs, and streamlining the computerized process for developing personalized retainers. The orthodontic maintenance regulations, which cover topics like retention adaptation issues, harmony along with maintaining a standard of proper dental hygiene, are managed by an artificial intelligence-powered program, called "Dental monitoring, Paris, France".(Khan et al., 2022)

The personalized nickel-titanium retainer can be computer-designed using a digital technology powered by AI with intraoral scanning of the teeth. The product is precisely manufactured through computer-aided design and computer-aided manufacturing (CAD-CAM) technology, ensuring a proper fit to the dental surfaces.(Cole et al., 2019)

The transparent plastic retainers are produced using three-dimensional printed designs derived from dental scans, and their precision is comparable to that made with conventional dental impressions.(Dietrich et al., 2017; Mohd Tahir et al., 2019)

1.3.20 Three dimensional (3D) printed orthodontic models

Study models in orthodontics can be developed via 3D printing because of its ease of use, precision, and visual analysis.(Lee et al., 2015b; Sherman et al., 2020).It can bypass the traditional process of obtaining impressions and casting procedures by turning a patient's digital model into an actual one.(Kim et al., 2018).Printed three-dimensional dental models have been enhanced by AI technology and can be used to make trays for indirect bonding, expanding devices, thermoplastic aligners, and removable appliances.(Martorelli et al., 2013)

1.3.21 Estimation of the treatment outcomes

AI plays a significant role in mimicking different clinical situations during assessment and treatment planning, enhancing precision and control while reducing clinical workload. Evaluating facial features is essential to orthodontics' examination and treatment strategy.

Artificial Neural Networks had been developed by (Nanda et al., 2015) to estimate variations in the curvature of the lip after treatment with or without extraction. The expected alteration for the upper lip was 29.6%, and for the lower lip, it was 7%.

Artificial neural networks have also been used by (Patcas et al., 2019), to evaluate the aesthetics of the face prior to and following orthognathic surgery using a rating system ranging from zero to one hundred. (Akçam and Takada, 2002), developed an automated simulation system to assist beginner orthodontists in selecting suitable headgear.

1.3.22 Temporary anchorage device (TAD) and mini plates placement using the surgical guide

Temporary anchorage devices (TADs) and mini plates are used for numerous orthodontic management modalities, such as those for "molar intrusion, open bite correction, molar distalization, and maxillary impaction or protraction". (Tsui et al., 2012).Therefore, their precise positioning is essential for successful treatment outcomes. The surgical guides' construction material should be sufficiently durable to maintain stabilization throughout the inserting process. Surgical guides created with 3D printing-powered AI modality have gained increasing popularity as they provide clinicians with a reliable and straightforward approach for the placement of TADs.(Al Mortadi et al., 2012; Al-Moghrabi et al., 2021).This offers appropriate adaptability, ensuring reliability and precision in the final placement of the TADs and mini plates. This approach guarantees optimal contact with the bone surface, enhancing security and reducing the likelihood of the TADs and mini plates loosening. (Salmi et al., 2012).

1.3.23 Robotic wire bending

An essential component of a therapeutic approach is the bending of orthodontic archwires.(Yongde et al., 2014).The efficiency regarding the traditional archwire bending procedure in wire manipulation depends on the specialist's ability level. The archwire requires multiple bends to achieve optimal treatment outcomes.(Jiang et al., 2015)

The "Bending Art System" is the first CAD/CAM technology created to produce personalized archwires. Researcher "Helge Fischer-Brandies" and his colleague developed the computer equipment with the programming in 1984 in collaboration with a technical company. It is applied in the fabrication of the labial and lingual archwires.(Aldrees, 2016)

This type of system includes an archwire bending machine and a bending device. The Suresmile program uses robotics-based digital technology for fabricating customized brackets and archwires. It uses modern software algorithms and three-dimensional photographic techniques for evaluation and planning procedures. A multi-component, AI-powered robotic framework is used in the "Cartesian-type archwire bending" (Figure 1.26) and (Figure 1.27). The bending mechanism is examined, and the archwire geometric configuration is developed using the appropriate program.(Jiang et al., 2016).When an automated device bends the archwire, the outcomes of orthodontic treatments will be much more successful, and the treatment will be notably faster.(Vaishnavi et al., 2021)

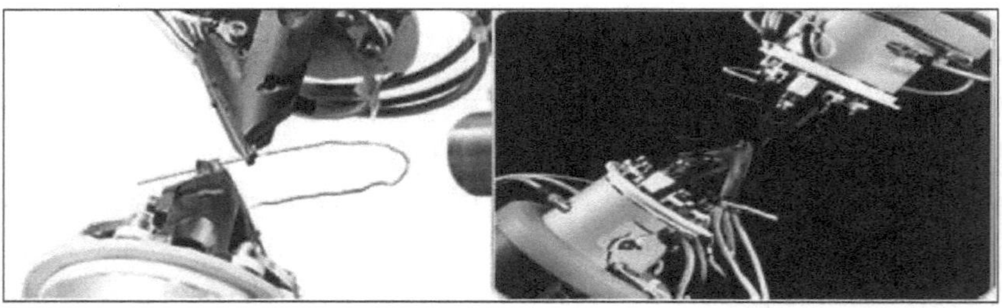

Figure 1.26: Suresmile orthodontic twisting archwire robots.(Abutayyem et al., 2019)

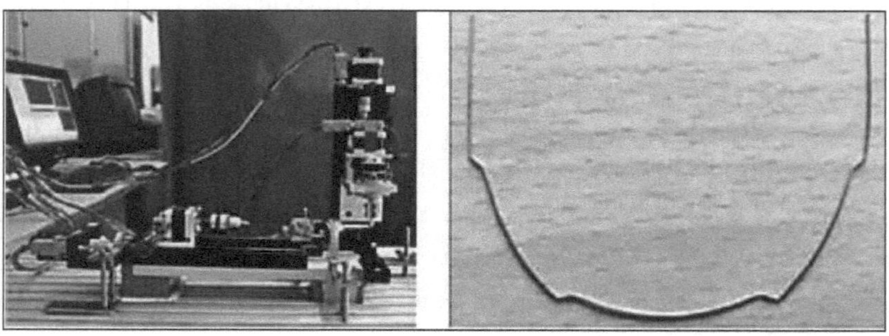

Figure 1.27: Orthodontic archwire bending robots that make the "Cartesian type bend".(Abutayyem et al., 2019)

1.3.24 Facial scan

Intelligent systems enhance face assessment beyond basic balance and ratios, providing a more thorough understanding of the anatomy of the face with its impact on oral health. It makes adapting therapeutic approaches to each patient's unique requirements easier. Additionally, artificial intelligence can customize equipment creation according to each patient in biomedical device development. Automated evaluation of facial features by artificial intelligence can identify unique facial traits in orthodontics and subsequently adjust treatment methods. Artificial intelligence systems in biomedicine analyze vast amounts of data to uncover correlations and improve system efficiency. This is also true for orthodontic face assessment technologies, which utilize individual data, including two-dimensional or three-dimensional facial scans, to offer treatment approach suggestions.(Goh et al., 2023)

Real maxillofacial assessments conducted with a caliper were compared to facial scans conducted by utilizing the "3D light scanner Artec Eva." The investigation demonstrated the high precision of the facial scanning workflow. However, the scanning method was required multiple times compared to direct maxillofacial assessment.(Franco de Sá Gomes et al., 2019)

1.4 Limitations and challenges of artificial intelligence

Artificial intelligence has shown substantial benefits across various scientific fields; however, its application in practice is fraught with challenges. Numerous difficulties may arise when employing artificial intelligence in dental care, particularly in orthodontic care.(Butul and Sharab, 2024).(Figure 1.28).

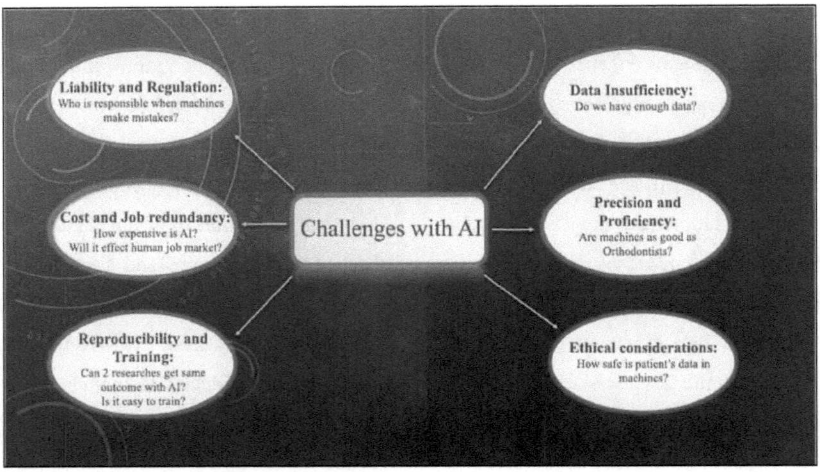

Figure 1.28: Primary concerns associated with the utilization of intelligent systems in orthodontics.(Butul and Sharab, 2024)

These concerns include:

1.4.1 Accuracy and Capabilities

Although artificial intelligence has been used to diagnose and plan treatments, evaluate cephalometric X-rays, and perform other tasks, it is essential to consider whether its capabilities match those of human professionals. Numerous investigations have shown that an orthodontic expert can treat challenging cases more accurately than artificial intelligence technologies.(Strunga et al., 2023)

Artificial intelligence may not be adaptable to unforeseen events, preferences of the patient, and various aspects like culture or faith, even when it provides rational options for therapy. Human involvement becomes essential to overcome these issues. Physician-patient interaction is greatly impeded by automated contact, which often lacks motivation.(Ayad et al., 2023)

According to multiple studies, patients favour physician-made recommendations for treatment over machine-made ones.(Promberger and Baron, 2006)

1.4.2 Job displacement and financial issues

Worries that artificial intelligence in medicine could eliminate professions have led to suspicion and resistance toward artificial intelligence projects. Profession replacement continues to be a significant issue of concern.(khan et al., 2023)

Skepticism regarding artificial intelligence prevents its wider use in the medical field. Raising the general knowledge of artificial intelligence for medical use is essential to resolving patient and physician viewpoints.(Cruciger et al., 2016; Díaz et al., 2019)

Significant resources are frequently required to create and maintain artificial intelligent technology, which may make them unavailable to a wide range of patients and medical professionals.(Strunga et al., 2023)

However, considering its capacity for streamlining the clinical workflow, several research investigations have proved artificial intelligence's economic aspect in contrast with conventional dentistry. However, to determine its usefulness in various contexts, additional investigations are necessary.(Schwendicke et al., 2021)

1.4.3 Ethical issues

While artificial intelligence augments human skills, it does not replace evaluating and developing treatment protocols. Getting patients' permission while clarifying the complicated functions of AI might be difficult. Regarding database marketing, the ethical preservation of patient confidentiality is essential. (Roganović et al., 2023)

Because of the recent development of intelligent systems and their usefulness in healthcare, achieving an equilibrium between resolving moral dilemmas and encouraging creativity is crucial. The concerns that need to be focused on when employing artificial intelligence in dentistry (Gerke et al., 2020):

1) Ensuring security and honesty
2) Obtaining permission for information utilization
3) Protecting the confidentiality of information
4) Addressing computational equity and biases

The technique and the final output are invisible since robots work independently, analyzing and drawing inferences from current information to create a fresh collection of information.(Roganović et al., 2023)

The public will have greater confidence among professionals as well as robots if issues of ethics are addressed. A questionnaire study revealed that 30% of the surveyed participants were worried that intelligent systems in healthcare would jeopardize the confidence bridge between individuals and physicians. (Ayad et al., 2023)

1.4.4 Insufficient database

The information used for modeling is essential for artificial intelligence, and it is crucial to consider selection bias when choosing a set of information. Several studies have shown that dental records, particularly those related to orthodontic treatment, often have a somewhat narrow scope. The potential for smaller datasets to yield automated outcomes that can be generalized to a larger community remains a topic of active discussion.(Butul and Sharab, 2024)

For instance, since those who visit university healthcare facilities are typically ill, data collected from colleges or universities may reflect a biased selection. Similarly, the dataset is derived from the wealthy population in societies without national insurance.(Gianfrancesco et al., 2018)

1.4.5 Practice and Reliable Performance

Every physician has a different point of view in a medical discussion. Likewise, achieving identical results from a system becomes difficult when two distinct investigators customize the algorithms. Inconsistencies among investigators and lacking technical and statistical skills have been attributed to these reliability issues.(Liu et al., 2021)

Familiarizing patients, students, and dental professionals with artificial intelligence is essential for its widespread adoption and for improving its reliability. When artificial intelligence is used correctly, physicians' responsibility decreases, and ethical standards are maintained.(Butul and Sharab, 2024)

1.4.6 Responsibility and Political Management

The capability of robots to achieve desired outcomes may become questionable as they adjust to new circumstances. There are no regulations in place that govern responsibility when artificial intelligence generates an unfair ethical outcome.(Martins, 2021).Companies should consider the responsibility issues if artificial intelligence does not meet expectations.(Dhopte and Bagde, 2023)

Dental professionals and orthodontic specialists need to understand artificial intelligence's limitations. They must also maintain accurate documentation and communicate honestly with patients about AI during their care. Preserving the confidentiality of health information is crucial to preventing the sale of medical data, which poses a significant issue due to the need for accurate information validation.(khan et al., 2023)

1.5 Up-to-date trends and future perspectives

AI advancements will enable individualized and patient-focused dental services in addition to improving the reliability and success of orthodontic examination and therapeutic approaches.(Tomášik et al., 2024).

1.5.1 AI up-to-date trends

- **Aesthetic assessment with facial analysis:** Facial-scanning programs supported by artificial intelligence evaluate facial proportion, harmony, and appearance. Orthodontic specialists are using this to develop more visually beautiful treatment strategies.
- **Orthodontic devices created using 3-D printing technology**: 3-D printing produces personalized orthodontic devices, including "aligners, retainers, and surgical guides". This enhances the convenience and fit of devices, streamlining management time and minimizing the necessity for adaptations.
- **Consistent patient follow-up**: An artificial intelligence-driven orthodontic evaluation program has been utilized to monitor patients' treatment progress and

identify potential relapse warning signs. This allows orthodontic professionals to act promptly and avoid potential treatment failures.

- **Artificial intelligence-driven analysis**: Systems are currently being created to streamline the examination of "cephalometric X-rays, 3D CBCT scans, and facial photographs." This will make treatment planning and implementation more effective by decreasing the efforts needed for conventional evaluation and analysis.

1.5.2 AI future perspectives

- **Individualized orthodontic procedures:** Artificial intelligence will develop customized procedures specific to each patient's objectives and requirements, making orthodontic procedures more personalized.
- **Visual treatment objectives:** VTO aims to enhance the orthodontic therapy process for patients through complete and dynamic approaches. This technology will enable patients to be more active in the diagnosis and treatment plan and better understand their medical care.
- **Enhancement of orthodontic treatment:** Artificial intelligence will improve the orthodontic treatment schedule, organization, and duration. This will lead to enhanced effectiveness and productivity in procedures.
- **Database for additional orthodontic investigation:** Artificial intelligence will analyze and assess comprehensive individual patient records to discover new ideas and develop more advanced treatment protocols. This will facilitate a greater awareness of the factors contributing to dental malocclusions and enhance the efficacy of therapeutic approaches.

1.6 Integrating intelligent systems into dental education

It is imperative to advance the dental profession by introducing artificial intelligence into the educational process. By developing specially designed programs and integrating detailed training in artificial intelligence into the academic curriculum, creative, reliable, and successful oral health care can be promoted. This change is inevitable; dental schools and other educational institutions should prepare future dentists to be just as competent in modern dentistry the same way they are in conventional treatment. (Dashti et al., 2024a)

1.6.1 Clinical Education

Artificial intelligence can be extremely beneficial in clinical dentistry training. It enhances healthcare by facilitating telecommuting through examining dental documents, the simulation of various potential scenarios, and the development of different designs. For instance, AI-powered software assists with examining and planning treatment protocols. These tools can aid clinicians in evaluating radiographs, dental scans, and images, acting as an extra set of hands to help them make more precise therapeutic decisions by instantly recognizing oral health concerns that may go unnoticed due to exhaustion, a heavy workload, or limited expertise, while also providing suggestions for organizing treatment. These programs enrich dental residents' and professionals' awareness and practical skills, which deliver more precise evaluations and plans for treatment. (Bayrakdar et al., 2023).(Figure 1.29)

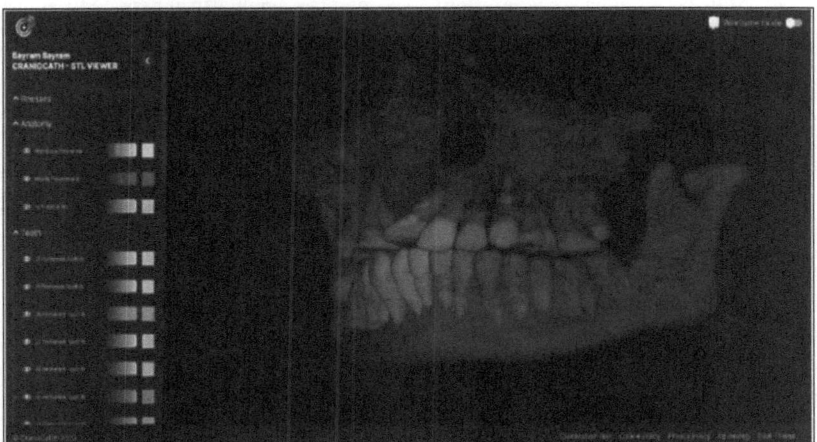

Figure 1.29: Automatic segmentation by "CranioCatch 3D.stl AI software" of a case scenario taken with cone beam computed tomography.(Bayrakdar et al., 2023)

1.6.2 Academic Education

In a study conducted by (Yüzbaşıoğlu, 2021) , assessed the "knowledge and attitudes of dental students toward AI and its possible application". Nearly 80% consensus exists that incorporating artificial intelligence is essential in undergraduate and higher education curricula.

It is increasingly evident that the core dentistry education program needs to be modified, and intelligent systems education must be incorporated in light of these improvements and dental student desires.(Bayrakdar et al., 2023)

A) Recommended academic guidelines

Educational organizations must create a thorough training system that covers the following to foster proficiency in artificial intelligence within dental education (Dashti et al., 2024a):

- **Different practical software workshops**: The training program should include hands-on exercises utilizing digital applications and artificial intelligence-driven diagnosis and designing programs.
- **Multidisciplinary cooperation:** To provide multidisciplinary educational experiences, dentistry colleges should work with technical colleges and scientific institutes to foster creativity in artificial intelligence implementation.
- **Teaching activities on ML and artificial intelligence:** Both fundamental and modern artificial intelligence principles, such as ML algorithms, dealing with data, and how they are employed in scanning, examination, and photography, should be covered during these sessions.

B) Necessity for more focused specialization in dentistry

Regarding the field of dental intelligent systems, there are currently no specialized master's or doctoral programs. The complete implementation of dental intelligent systems is hindered by this academic gap, which in turn limits the development of novel innovations specifically suited to medical treatment. Courses that carefully investigate artificial intelligence's possible uses in dentistry and provide instruction on the profession's basic concepts are essential. Medical professionals in the future will be able to quickly adjust to revolutionary technological devices and develop innovative ways to enhance patient care, as such programs will equip them with the necessary skills to do so.(Dashti et al., 2024b)

C) Main limitations and concerns

There are multiple challenges associated with incorporating intelligent systems into school programs:(Dashti et al., 2024a)

1) Substantial funding is needed to build facilities, purchase modern machines, and educate teachers.
2) Regularly revising course materials to reflect new knowledge and skills gained through continuous innovations is essential.
3) Strict attention must be given to ethical concerns, especially the confidentiality of clinical records and the accuracy of artificial intelligence judgments made in healthcare contexts.
4) Both academics and professionals in the field need to be knowledgeable about these challenges to employ AI successfully and ethically.

D) Encouragement of proactive steps

The following steps are essential for future academic progress (Dashti et al., 2024a) :

- A combined effort from colleges and universities, lawmakers, and company managers is necessary to overcome all possible obstacles and utilize artificial intelligence in dentistry to its fullest potential.
- To keep up with the latest innovations in dentistry teaching and research, educational institutions should work towards creating artificial intelligence courses and forming collaborations with IT organizations.
- Federations representing dentists must advocate for rules that explicitly outline how the profession should address the moral implications of artificial intelligence.

MATERIALS AND METHODS

2.1 Study design and sampling approach

A cross-sectional study has been performed involving orthodontists throughout Iraq. The aim was to assess their knowledge, awareness, and attitudes toward dental artificial intelligence and its potential applications in orthodontics.

The inclusion criteria included academicians and clinicians with higher education qualifications affiliated with the accredited Iraqi Orthodontic Society (IOS), while the exclusion criteria consisted of certified orthodontists, orthodontic residents, and general dental practitioners.

To ascertain the appropriate survey completion time, the surveylength.com.lnk tool was applied according to the percentage of respondents by questionnaire paths and respondents' age, in addition to the type and number of questions, with the word count of the paragraphs mentioned in the very first section of the Google form ahead of the questionnaire items. The estimated time to complete the survey was five minutes and eleven seconds. The recommended time to achieve a good response rate is five to ten minutes.

The total number of survey respondents was divided by the number of contacted and addressed IOS members to determine the response rate (currently, the IOS has 160 registered Iraqi orthodontists in its records).

2.2 Questionnaire development, design, and validation

2.2.1 Step number one: - Questions development by the researcher

The researcher created a pool of questions after conducting a comprehensive evaluation of several previous studies about the perception, knowledge, training, and applications regarding artificial intelligence in practical clinical dentistry procedures.(Aboalshamat, 2022; Lin et al., 2023; Pringle et al., 2024; Jeong et al., 2024; Mengi et al., 2024; Hanenkrath et al., 2025) .In addition to the raised issues regarding the contemporary era of dental artificial intelligence.

2.2.2 Step number two: - Questions development in consultation with six orthodontic experts

Six qualified orthodontic experts were invited to provide their insights on the key questions and items to be incorporated into the survey, aiming to address the most relevant aspects and highlight major concerns regarding dental AI in orthodontic practice in Iraq. All these experts were academicians with PhD qualifications in orthodontics, working in four different and well-recognized universities in Iraq, with varying levels of clinical experience (more than ten years) and from diverse geographical areas (Table 2.1).

Table 2. 1: Specialization and institutional affiliation of experts for survey development and content validation

Expert Code	Academic affiliation	Years of academic and clinical experience in orthodontics
Expert number one	Orthodontic Department /College of Dentistry - Baghdad University	18 years
Expert number two	Orthodontic Department /College of Dentistry - Mosul University	20 years
Expert number three	Orthodontic Department /College of Dentistry - University of Sulaimani	17 years
Expert number four	Orthodontic Department /College of Dentistry – University of Sulaimani	18 years
Expert number five	Orthodontic Department /College of Dentistry - Hawler Medical University	17 years
Expert number six	Orthodontic Department /College of Dentistry - Hawler Medical University	12 years

After the expert panel granted approval for participation, a Zoom meeting was conducted to provide them with comprehensive information regarding the aim of the questionnaire, the target survey group, the development and design process, and the upcoming content validation procedures. This ensured that they were well informed, had a precise understanding, and were fully aware of all the necessary details to develop carefully structured and valid survey items in line with (Waltz et al., 1991; Davis, 1992).

All opinions and items submitted by experts for inclusion in the survey were carefully reviewed and analyzed by the researcher, and only those deemed necessary were considered. The initial draft of the survey instrument included 29 closed-ended questions, including those developed by the researcher and those developed in consultation with orthodontic experts.

(Figure 2.1) outlines the phases of the expert panel assessment procedure, starting by the survey's initial version, then culminating in the review stage. In cases where the items are revised based on experts' feedback, the revised survey should be re-evaluated by the same procedures with experts in subsequent rounds.(Davis, 1992)

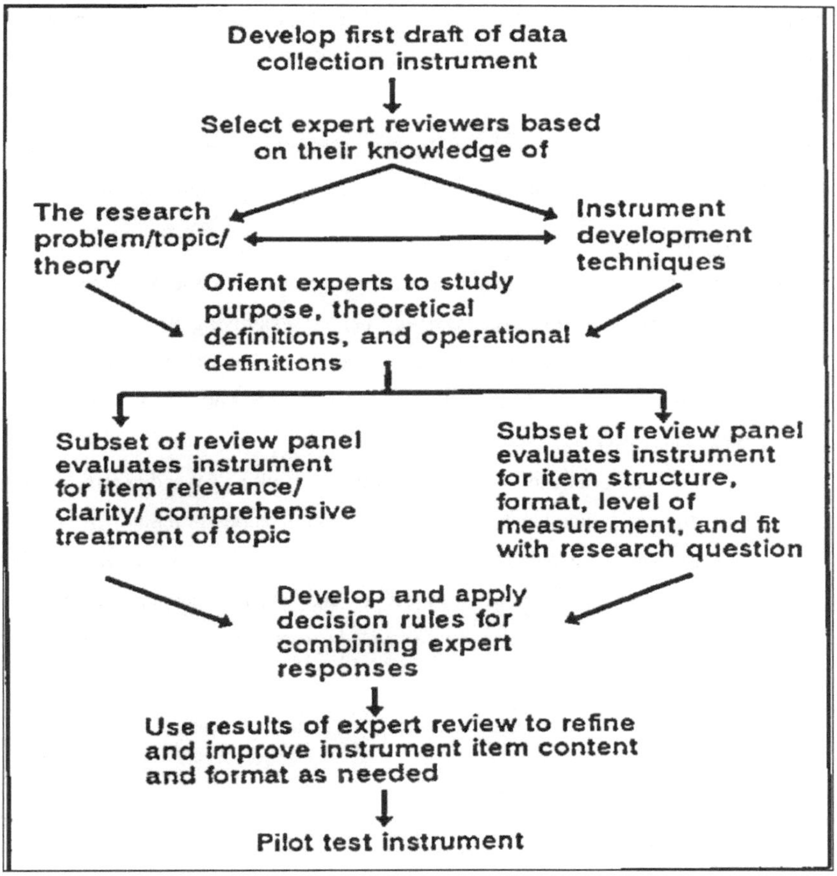

Figure 2. 1: Survey evaluation stages.(Davis, 1992)

2.2.3 Step number three: Questionnaire validation

An expert panel for content and face validation evaluated the survey instrument.

Validation refers to the questionnaire's potential to achieve its goals, specifically whether it accurately assesses what is intended to be evaluated.(Yassir et al., 2016)

Content validation represents the extent to which the questionnaire components are pertinent and represent the key ideas in the context of the assessment's specific purpose. (Haynes et al., 1995)

(Lynn, 1986) Characterized content validity as a thorough evaluation, staging two parts, "construction and evaluation steps ", essential to nearly every assessment in the survey instrument.

- Construction step: Evaluation of content validation starts at the very early stage of survey creation. It includes three key phases: identifying the research scope, developing items, and structuring the survey instrument. (Carmines and Zeller, 1979; Williamson, 1981; DeVellis, 1991; Gable and Wolf, 1993; Nunnally and Bernstein, 1994)
- The next is the evaluation step, which involves consulting defined experts to assess the validity of individual items and the overall survey validity.(Lynn, 1986; DeVellis, 1991; Gable and Wolf, 1993).This step is undertaken to determine if the survey items suit the research objectives and whether any items need to be eliminated or more items need to be added.(Lynn, 1986; Polit and Beck, 2004; Schultz and Whitney, 2005).

2.3 Validation types and procedures

2.3.1 Content validity procedure

The survey items were validated for their content in two phases using the content validity ratio (CVR) and content validity index (CVI) according to Lawshe's method.

This method has been widely adopted in academic studies, medical research, organizational improvement, and similar fields. The Lawshe method's key strengths over other methods are its clarity, ease of use, straightforward calculation, and support by predefined tables to identify the critical CVR values accurately. (Wilson et al., 2012)

The global recognition of Lawshe's method among research professionals is largely due to its precision and focused nature. It ranks and prioritizes items based on the assessments of qualified experts. Furthermore, studies confirm that content validity ratio analysis can identify relevant items through analytical evaluation.(Samad et al., 2023). Procedures for establishing content validity include the following:

A) Expert panel for content validation

The panel of experts involved is usually determined by the availability and willingness of suitable candidates that the researcher can find, rather than relying on population estimation guidelines.

- A group of at least five experts is usually sufficient to prevent random agreement from influencing the results.
- In fields where locating qualified experts is challenging, a panel of three experts is adequate. However, a group of (five to ten experts) is typically recommended, while exceeding ten experts is generally unwarranted. (Lynn, 1986)

For this research study, the same six orthodontic experts (Table 2.1) were invited again to proceed with the content validity procedure. These experts were purposefully selected for their extensive experience in the field, with many published papers on AI in orthodontics. They have actively participated in many regional and international conferences related to AI, posing a deep understanding of AI applications in orthodontics, and have integrated various AI-powered tools and software into their clinical orthodontic practice.

The recruitment of these experts was based on the "Standards for Educational and Intellectual Evaluation by the American Educational Research Association, American Psychological Association, & National Council on Measurement in Education, 1985," which recommended that the selection of the expert panel be guided by their expertise, specialized training, and competence. A valuable criterion for selecting these experts includes their presentation at national conferences, conducting academic studies on the relevant topic with a history of publishing in respected journals, as indicated by (Grant and Kinney, 1992).

B) Content validity assessment form

This form is structured into four parts (Appendix I, the content validity assessment form, included the invitation letter and the initial draft of the survey). The first part presented a cover letter outlining the survey's title, researchers' names, qualifications, affiliations, and email addresses, along with a clear note stating that participation is voluntary. It also assured the participating experts that their submitted responses would be kept confidential.

Next was the content validation section, which highlighted the aim of the invitation, the purpose of the questionnaire, and clear guidelines for assessing the accuracy and thoroughness of the items to gather "evidence-based items" for possible incorporation in the final survey, and eliminating any non-essential items that aren't related to the domain being investigated.(Oluwatayo, 2012; Elangovan and Sundaravel, 2021).Experts' evaluations are what ultimately decide the content validity.

The subsequent third section of the form for assessing the content validity included the instrument rating sheet, which detailed the survey sections along with their corresponding questions, a column for each point on a scale, and dedicated side columns for experts to provide suggestions, propose improvements, highlight items needing refinement, and identify any potential deficiencies as recommended by (Lynn, 1986).

Every expert was tasked to independently assess the essentiality level for every survey question according to a rating scale with three points, as indicated by (Lawshe, 1975):

- Scale No.1 ➔ "Essential"
- Scale No.2 ➔ "Useful but not essential"
- Scale No.3 ➔ "Not necessary"

The final section of the form included a copy of the survey questions' original draft. The researchers shared the content validity assessment form with every assigned expert. Then, the feedback from each expert was received without further intervention or discussion and kept confidential from other experts.

C) Computing the content validity ratio (CVR)

The content validity ratio is a well-established index that supports decisions about accepting or rejecting items within the survey instrument. This approach is widely acknowledged as a means of establishing the validity of content.(Wilson et al., 2012)

We can definitely choose whether to retain or remove an item when all or none of the experts evaluate the assessed subject or information as 'essential'. Challenges emerge in the absence of a unified agreement. (Gilbert and Prion, 2016)

Two suppositions are proposed by (Lawshe, 1975) :-

- A certain level of content validity is assumed when an item receives over fifty percent of the experts' "essential" ratings.
- A greater percentage of content validity is indicated by an item's rating as "Essential" by a larger number of experts (above the 50% threshold).

The following equation was used to calculate the content validity ratio for each of the items (Lawshe, 1975):

$$CVR = \frac{N_e - (\frac{N}{2})}{N/2}$$

In which: -

Ne = Is the count of experts who gave an item the "Essential" rating.

N = Is the overall count of specialists (where N/2 represents only half of that amount).

The following are the potential outcomes for the content validity ratio, ranging from (-1 to +1):

- The item is considered crucial and would be incorporated into the survey when all professionals assess it as "Essential", meaning the CVR score equals to +1 (for more straightforward computation, it is adjusted to 0.99).

- If the CVR score is negative and getting close to -1 (CVR <0), it indicates an item was assessed as "Essential" by fewer than half of the professionals, and that item should be excluded from the question pool.
- In situations where more than 50% of professionals rated an item as "Essential," but not all did, the CVR score falls between "0 and 0.99."
- When 50% of professionals consider an item to be "Essential" and 50% do not, the CVR score is zero (CVR=0).

Retention or exclusion of the questions from the survey's question pool was based on the CVR values, which are decided by the number of panelists involved in the study, as indicated in (Table 2.2).

Table 2. 2: CVR minimum values, P=0.05 (Lawshe, 1975)

No. of Panelists	Min. Value*
5	.99
6	.99
7	.99
8	.75
9	.78
10	.62
11	.59
12	.56
13	.54
14	.51
15	.49
20	.42
25	.37
30	.33
35	.31
40	.29

(Table 2.2) displays the minimum CVR values calculated according to the number of panelists. A total of six orthodontic experts participated in this research project.

D) Calculating the content validity index (CVI)

The CVI value is the calculated mean of all items retained in the final survey instrument. (DeVon et al., 2007).CVI is measured to determine the overall questionnaire's validity.

- A content validity index value of 0.70 is reasonable.(Tilden et al., 1990)
- (Davis, 1992), recommended a CVI value of more than 0.80 for newly developed survey instruments.
- (Waltz, 2005) , suggested that a CVI threshold of 0.90 and above is regarded as acceptable and indicative of perfect content validity.
- A low CVI score may signify that the survey instrument has issues with survey development and item quality, incorrect expert recruitment for validation, or potential bias from the experts themselves. Additionally, it could stem from inadequate guidance and information provided to the expert panel.(Polit et al., 2007).

E) Stages of assessing the content validation by six orthodontic experts for this questionnaire study.

1) Stage number one: Results of the CVR (Content validity ratio for each item) and the CVI (Content validity index for the overall questionnaire) in the first content validation phase.

According to the results of CVR, which provides validity per every question individually, questions with a CVR score equal to 1 have been considered "valid" and included in the survey's question pool. Others were either "rejected" or "refined according to the suggestions and recommendations provided by the experts".

The analysis showed that (Table 2.3): -

- Eleven items obtained full approval (CVR=1) and were rated essential by all experts. The decision was made to incorporate these items into the final survey's draft.

- Fifteen items were rated essential (CVR=0.67) by just five experts. A total of twelve questions underwent revisions in response to the suggestions and instructions offered by the experts' feedback, and three items were given serious consideration for retention in the survey instrument, owing to their contribution as relevant items.
- Three items achieved a CVR value of zero, which is under the established value. These items were excluded from the question pool.
- The questionnaire's overall CVI was 0.72, which does not meet the recommended threshold for validation.

Table 2. 3 : Results of content validity ratio for each item and content validity index for the overall questionnaire in the first content validation phase by six orthodontic experts

Main Sections	**NO. Of the question**	**Survey Questions**	**Number of specialists ranked an item as Essential "Ne"**	**CVR**	**Researchers' analysis and decisions are guided by experts' feedback.**	**CVI**
1. Demographic data and professional background	Q1	What is your gender?	6	1	**Valid/ Accepted**	**0.72**
	Q2	How old are you?	5	0.67	**Refined**	
	Q3	What is your academic achievement?	6	1	**Valid/ Accepted**	
	Q4	How many years of clinical	5	0.67	**Refined**	

		experience do you have?				
	Q5	Which institution do you belong to?	6	1	**Valid/ Accepted**	
	Q6	What is your main region of residency?	6	1	**Valid/ Accepted**	
2. Knowledge and awareness of AI	Q1	How did you hear about AI applications that are certainly designed for orthodontics?	5	0.67	**Refined**	
	Q2	How would you evaluate your scientific knowledge about AI in orthodontics?	3	0	**Not valid/ Excluded**	
	Q3	Which AI orthodontic software have you used?	5	0.67	**Retained**	
3. Perception about the use	Q1	Are you aware of the use of	5	0.67	**Refined**	

of AI in orthodontic practice		AI-powered software programs for diagnosis and treatment planning in orthodontic practice?				
	Q2	Are you aware of the utilization of AI in digitization and lateral cephalometric analysis?	5	0.67	**Refined**	
	Q3	Are you aware of AI's role in preparing and planning for orthognathic surgery/Corre-cting facial aesthetics?	5	0.67	**Refined**	
	Q4	In your opinion, is the diagnosis and treatment	6	1	**Valid / Accepted**	

		planning of AI-powered software better than that of an experienced human orthodontist?				
4. Attitudes about the use of AI in orthodontics	Q1	Are you currently using AI-powered tools in your orthodontic practice?	6	1	**Valid/ Accepted**	
	Q2	Which type of activity do you use AI for in your practice?	3	0	**Not valid/ Excluded**	
	Q3	If the clinical decision differs from the artificial intelligence decision, which one do you trust?	5	0.67	**Refined**	

	Q4	Are you aware of using AI-assisted tools like the prediction of canine impaction, determination of the geometry of orthodontic spring with force to align the teeth, and software to select the suitable headgear?	5	0.67	**Refined**	
	Q5	In which area of orthodontics do you think AI will be promising?	5	0.67	**Refined**	
	Q6	Do you find that AI-assisted orthodontics saves time for diagnosis and	5	0.67	**Refined**	

		treatment planning?				
	Q7	Do you agree that AI-assisted orthodontics will boost treatment costs?	3	0	**Not valid/ Excluded**	
	Q8	Would you be interested in receiving formal training on AI in orthodontics and integrating AI-based tools into your practice?	5	0.67	**Retained**	
5. Impact of dental AI in orthodontic practice	Q1	How has AI impacted your clinical decision-making process during orthodontic diagnosis and treatment planning?	6	1	**Valid/ Accepted**	

	Q2	Rate the impact of dental AI on the following aspects of orthodontics	6	1	**Valid/ Accepted**	
	Q3	Do you agree that the use of AI would improve the treatment quality and accuracy in orthodontics?	6	1	**Valid/ Accepted**	
6. Challenges, limitations, and future of AI in orthodontics	Q1	What do you think are the biggest challenges in adopting AI in Orthodontics?	6	1	**Valid/ Accepted**	
	Q2	Do you believe artificial intelligence could substitute orthodontists in clinical practice?	5	0.67	**Retained**	

	Q3	Do you believe orthodontists can base on AI-powered programs as a second judgment in complex cases for diagnosis and treatment in the near future?	5	0.67	**Refined**	
	Q4	Do you think AI will play a significant role in the future of orthodontic practice in Iraq?	6	1	**Valid/ Accepted**	
	Q5	Do you believe AI-related education training should be included in undergraduate and postgraduate orthodontic curriculum?	5	0.67	**Refined**	

2) Stage number two: Questionnaire adjustments following the first content validation phase.

The questionnaire was updated as detailed below: -

A) Excluding three invalid items, namely (item **No. 2 in section 2, item No. 2, and item No. 7 in section 4**).

B) Modifying the following items to express more precision and clarity: -

1. **Item No.2 in section 1** was converted from (How old are you) to (What is your year of birth?).
2. **Item No.4 in section 1** was modified from (How many years of clinical experience do you have?) to (How many years of clinical experience do you have in orthodontics?).
3. **Item No. 1 in Section 2** was converted from (How did you hear about AI applications that are certainly designed for orthodontics?) to (How did you learn about AI software programs specifically designed for orthodontics?), and one additional option was added to the multiple choices which is (Web browsing such as Google advertisements, Internet Explorer, YouTube advertisements, etc.).
4. **Item No.5 in section 4** was modified from (In which area of orthodontics do you think AI will be promising?) to (In which area of orthodontics would you apply AI if its results prove to be promising?), and two additional options were added to the multiple choices which are (Practice management) and (patient's education and communication).
5. **Item No.3 in section 6** was changed from (Do you believe orthodontists can base on AI-powered programs as a second judgment in complex cases for diagnosis and treatment in the near future ?) to (Do you believe orthodontists could rely on AI-powered programs as a secondary tool for judgment in complex cases for diagnosis and treatment planning in the near future?).
6. **Item No.5 in section 6** was converted from (Do you believe AI-related education training should be included in the undergraduate and postgraduate orthodontic curriculum?) to (Do you recommend including AI-related education training in undergraduate and postgraduate orthodontic curricula?).

C) Reorganizing the following items between the sections to enhance their relevance in terms of meaning and logical linkage: -

1. Shifting items **No.1** (Are you aware of using AI-powered software programs for diagnosis and treatment planning in orthodontic practice?), **No.2** (Are you aware of the use of AI in digitization and lateral cephalometric analysis?), and **No.3** (Are you aware of AI's role in the preparation and planning of orthognathic surgery or in correcting facial aesthetics?) from section **No. 3** to section **No. 2.**
2. Shifting item **No.4** (Are you aware of using AI-assisted tools like the prediction of canine impaction, determination of the geometry of orthodontic spring with force to align the teeth, and software to select the suitable headgear?) from section **No. 4** to section **No. 2.**
3. Shifting items **No.3** (If the clinical decision differs from the artificial intelligence decision, which one do you trust?) and **No.6** (Do you find that AI-assisted orthodontics saves time for diagnosis and treatment planning?) from section **No. 4** to section **No. 3.**

D) The following three items, rated essential by five experts (CVR = 0.67), were carefully reviewed for inclusion in the survey instrument due to their relevance and significance, namely: -

1. **Item No. 3 in section No. 2**, following the adjustment and reorganization, became question No. 2 in the same section.
2. **Item No. 8 in section No. 4**, following the adjustment and reorganization, became question No. 3 in the same section.
3. **Item No. 2 in section No. 6**

3) Stage number three: Results of the CVR (Content validity ratio for each refined item) and the CVI (Content validity index for the overall questionnaire) in the second content validation phase.

In the second content validation phase, the same six orthodontic expert panels were invited again to evaluate questionnaire updates and adjustments after three-week intervals following the first content validation phase, as recommended by (Lynn, 1986). The twelve refined items were rated as "Essential" (CVR=1), and the content validity index of the overall questionnaire was (CVI=0.96), which indicates perfect agreement and roughly excellent content validity (Table 2.4).

Table 2. 4 : CVR and CVI results for the second content validation phase.

Main Section	**NO. Of the question**	**Survey questions**	**Types of refinement and adjustments**	**CVR**	**Result**	**CVI**
1. Demographic data and professional background	Q2	What is your year of birth?	Modified	1	**Valid**	**0.96**
	Q4	How many years of clinical experience do you have in orthodontics?	Modified	1	**Valid**	
2. Knowledge and awareness of AI	Q1	How did you learn about AI software programs specifically	Modified, and an additional option was added to the	1	**Valid**	

		designed for orthodontics?	multiple choices.			
	Q3	Are you aware of using AI-powered software programs for diagnosis and treatment planning in orthodontic practice?	Shifted from Section No. 3	1	**Valid**	
	Q4	Are you aware of the use of AI in digitization and lateral cephalometric analysis?	Shifted from section No. 3	1	**Valid**	
	Q5	Are you aware of AI's role in the preparation and planning of orthognathic surgery or in correcting	Shifted from section No. 3	1	**Valid**	

		facial aesthetics?				
	Q6	Are you aware of using AI-assisted tools like the prediction of canine impaction, determination of the geometry of orthodontic spring with force to align the teeth, and software to select the suitable headgear?	Shifted from section No. 4	1	**Valid**	
3. Perception about the use of AI in Orthodontic practice	Q1	Do you find that AI-assisted orthodontics saves time for diagnosis and treatment planning?	Shifted from section No. 4	1	**Valid**	

	Q2	If the clinical decision differs from the artificial intelligence decision, which one do you trust?	Shifted from section No. 4	1	**Valid**	
4. Attitudes about the use of AI in Orthodontics	Q2	In which area of orthodontics would you apply AI if its results prove to be promising?	Modified, and two additional options were added to the multiple choices.	1	**Valid**	
6. The Challenges, limitations, and future of AI in orthodontics	Q3	Do you believe orthodontists could rely on AI-powered programs as a secondary tool for judgment in complex cases for diagnosis and	Modified	1	**Valid**	

		treatment planning in the near future?				
	Q5	Do you recommend including AI-related education training in undergraduate and postgraduate orthodontic curricula?	Modified	1	**Valid**	

2.3.2 Face validity procedures

Face validation involves subjective evaluation of the survey items, ensuring they are feasible, readable, well-formatted, stylistically appropriate, and evident in language. This allows respondents to understand and answer the questions without ambiguity.(Oluwatayo, 2012).Including face and content validation is essential to verify that the questionnaire assesses its intended objectives. (Al-Naseri, 2017).

The face validity of this survey instrument was assessed by measuring inter-rater reliability using percent agreement and the Cohen kappa index (CKI).

Reliability is a key factor in establishing the credibility of study quality, results, and ultimate outcomes. Ensuring rater reliability is essential because it indicates the degree to which the study's data truly reflects the measured variables. Inter-rater reliability assesses the level of agreement among raters. It measures the degree to which different raters consistently assign identical scores to the given variables.(McHugh, 2012)

The steps for face validity procedures included the following:

A) Expert Panel for face validation

Two orthodontic experts were appointed and invited to assess the face validity of this questionnaire. Both experts were academicians at the College of Dentistry/Hawler Medical University, with over ten years of experience in the clinical and educational fields. (Table 2.5).

Table 2. 5: Expert panel for face validation

Expert code	Qualification	Academic affiliation	Years of academic and clinical experience in orthodontics
Expert number one	PhD in orthodontics	Senior specialist at “Orthodontic Department/College of Dentistry-Hawler Medical University”	17 years

Expert number two	MSc in orthodontics	Senior specialist at "Orthodontic Department/College of Dentistry-Hawler Medical University"	17 years

B) Face validity assessment form

The face validity assessment form is designed like the content validity assessment form (Appendix II, the invitation letter, face validity assessment form, and the survey questions draft after content validation). The first section included a cover letter outlining the survey's title, the researchers' names, qualifications, affiliations, and email addresses. The participating experts were assured that their submitted responses would remain confidential and be used solely for research purposes.

The second section pointed out the aim of the invitation, the purpose of the questionnaire, and detailed guidelines for evaluating the effectiveness of the survey instrument and assessing how well it meets its intended application. The specialists were instructed to evaluate the face validity based on the following seven criteria by (Oluwatayo , 2012) :-

1) Consistency and relevance of items to the survey's perceived goal.
2) Suitability of the layout.
3) Appropriateness of language difficulty concerning the respondents' level of knowledge.
4) Proper text font size and line spacing.
5) Spelling accuracy of complex terms.
6) The transparency and clear meaning of items.
7) Accurate and suitable grammatical usage.

The third section included the face validity rating form. The expert panel was asked to provide independent ratings using a dichotomous scale of 'Yes' (agree) and 'No' (disagree) for each of the seven criteria mentioned above. The agreement score indicates that the questions are consistently organized and categorized favorably within the appropriate topic group (Sangoseni et al., 2013).

Additionally, the experts were asked to share their perspectives, comments, and suggestions for further improvement of the survey items in the subsequent fourth section. The final part included an attached copy of the survey questions following content validation.

C) Results of assessment for face validation by two orthodontic experts

Responses from both experts were analyzed. (Table 2.6) shows the expert panel assessment for face validity. The evaluation results for the seven criteria by two experts showed that their assessments were identical for six criteria, with a difference in their evaluation in only one criterion (criterion No.7).

Both experts recommended modifying the layout by optimizing text size and line spacing to enhance readability. Additionally, both suggested adjusting the language of certain items to be more user-friendly and aligned with the recipient's comprehension level and language ability. Expert No.1 advised modifying the grammar of some questions.

Table 2. 6: Results of the expert panel assessment for the face validation with the calculated percent agreement and Cohen's kappa index.

Assessment criteria	Expert number one	Expert number two
1)Consistency and relevance of items to the survey's perceived goal.	Yes	Yes
2) Suitability of the layout.	No	No
3)Appropriateness of language difficulty concerning the respondents' level of knowledge.	Yes	Yes
4)Proper text font size and line spacing	No	No
5)Spelling accuracy of complex terms.	Yes	Yes
6)The transparency and clear meaning of items	No	No

7)Accurate and suitable grammatical usage.	No	Yes
Overall agreement	(6/7, six out of seven criteria)	
Percent agreement		85 %
Cohen's kappa index		0.72

D) Computing the percent agreement and Cohen's kappa index for face validation

1) Percent agreement

Percent agreement (observed agreement) was calculated using an Excel workbook to determine the agreement rate between both raters (experts). A table was created where the columns represent the raters and the rows indicate the variables (seven assessment criteria) for which the experts recorded their ratings.

The values have been recorded as 0 (for disagreements) and 1 (for agreements). Percent agreement was performed by subtracting Expert No. 2's scores from Expert No. 1's scores, then counting the number of zeros, and dividing it by the total number of variables.(McHugh, 2012)

The difference between both raters was zero for six criteria (criterion No. 1-criterion No. 6) except for criterion No.7; the difference was one score. In conclusion, there were six agreements, and the percentage was 85%. (Table 2.7)

Table 2. 7 : Results of the percent agreement for face validation

Assessment Criteria	Expert number one	Expert number two	Difference (Inter-rater agreement)
1)Consistency and relevance of items to the survey's perceived goal	1	1	0
2) Suitability of the layout.	0	0	0
3)Appropriateness of language difficulty concerning the respondents' level of knowledge	1	1	0
4)Proper text font size and line spacing	0	0	0
5)Spelling accuracy of complex terms.	1	1	0
6)The transparency and clear meaning of items	0	0	0
7)Accurate and suitable grammatical usage.	0	1	-1
Number of 0			**6**
Total number of criteria			**7**
Percent agreement (Inter-rater reliability)			**0.85**

Percent agreement is considered a conventional rater agreement analysis. The advantage of (percent agreement statistics) is that it is computationally simple and offers a straightforward interpretation. Still, its major drawback is that it fails to account for the chance that raters are guessing their scores, potentially inflating the actual agreement.(McHugh, 2012)

In the 1960s, Jacob Cohen, a renowned statistician, introduced Cohen's Kappa as a key metric for evaluating inter-rater reliability. He emphasized that when raters are uncertain about the right decision and guess, there is likely to be a certain amount of agreement between them. The key strength of Cohen's Kappa statistics is that it accounts for agreement among raters that occurs by chance, excluding any chance-related factors.(Cohen, 1960)

(McHugh, 2012) declared that "Perhaps the best advice for researchers is to calculate both percent agreement and kappa. If there is likely to be much guessing among the raters, it may make sense to use the kappa statistic, but if raters are well trained and little guessing is likely to exist, the researcher may safely rely on percent agreement to determine interrater reliability".

From this perspective, although the raters chosen for this study were highly experienced and carefully selected and instructed, the Cohen's kappa statistic was also included.

2) Cohen's Kappa Index

Cohen's kappa measures the potential for raters to make uncertain guesses on specific variables.

A kappa score falls between -1 and +1.(McHugh, 2012).Interpretation of Cohen's kappa values according to (Masuwai et al., 2024) :-

- Absolute agreement among assessors is indicated by a Cohen's kappa score of +1.
- A Cohen's kappa score of -1 demonstrates no agreement among the assessors.
- A Cohen's kappa value of 0 signifies no association between the assessments of both examiners.
- Kappa values of (0.60-0.79) are considered significant.

Kappa values lower than 0.60 indicate insufficient agreement between both raters, reducing the confidence in the accuracy of the study outcomes.(McHugh, 2012)

For this research study, Cohen's kappa was computed using DATAtab software. (Table 2.8)

Table 2. 8 : Results of Cohen's kappa

Cohen's kappa	P-value
0.72	.005

- **Cohen's kappa**

The kappa value was equal to 0.72, which suggests a substantial level of agreement among raters beyond what was expected by chance. It indicates that both raters were substantially more consistent in their assessments than if they had made their ratings randomly.

- **P value**

A p-value of (0.005) is below the conventional threshold of 0.05, indicating that the level of agreement (Kappa = 0.72) is statistically significantly different from (zero), and there is a low probability that the observed agreement is due to random chance.

In conclusion, and as indicated by (Altman, 1999) (Table 2.9), a kappa value of 0.72 reflects (a good strength of agreement beyond chance) and, therefore, an adequate level of validity, confirming the reliability of survey items for data collection.

Table 2. 9 : Altman's interpretation of Cohen's kappa values. (Altman, 1999)

Value of κ	Strength of agreement
< 0.20	Poor
0.21–0.40	Fair
0.41–0.60	Moderate
0.61–0.80	Good
0.81–1.00	Very good

*Note: k=kappa

E) Revision of the questionnaire items after face validation

The experts proposed modifications to the format and layout of some items. All experts' inputs have been reviewed and evaluated, and the items have been revised as listed below:-

- Items **No. 3, No. 5, and No. 6** in **section No. 1** were updated to (What is your highest academic qualification?), (Which institution are you affiliated with?), and (What is your region of residence?), respectively.
- Item **No. 6** in **section No. 2** was modified to (Are you familiar with using AI-assisted tools, such as predicting canine impaction, determining the geometry of orthodontic springs used to apply force for teeth alignment, and software for selecting the appropriate headgear?).
- Items **No. 1** and **No. 3** in **section No. 3** were updated to (Do you believe that AI-assisted orthodontics helps save diagnosis and treatment planning time?) and (Do you believe the diagnosis and treatment planning provided by AI-powered software are superior to those of an experienced orthodontist?), respectively.

- Item **No. 1** in **section No. 5** was modified to (To what extent has AI impacted your clinical decision-making process during orthodontic diagnosis and treatment planning?).
- Item **No. 1** in **section No. 6** was updated to (What do you consider to be the biggest challenges in adopting AI in orthodontics?).

Before the official release, a panel of five orthodontic specialists from the orthodontic department at Hawler Medical University's College of Dentistry reviewed the finalized questionnaire to identify any necessary edits or improvements.

The final version of the validated questionnaire consisted of 25 closed-ended questions and one open-ended question distributed across six sections (Appendix III, survey sections and questions after content and face validation), as outlined below: -

- The first section involved five closed-ended single-choice items (Q1, Q3, Q4, Q5, and Q6) and one open-ended question (Q2) about the respondents' demographic information and professional background.
- The second section, with six items, two multiple-choice items (Q1 and Q2) and four single-choice items (Q3-Q6), aimed to evaluate participants' fundamental knowledge and awareness of dental artificial intelligence use and application in orthodontics.
- The third section featured three single-choice items that focused on specialists' perceptions of utilizing AI in their clinical orthodontic practice and the effectiveness of AI-assisted diagnosis and treatment planning.
- Questions about participants' attitudes were emphasized in the fourth section, which included three items: one Likert-scale item (Q1) assesses the extent of respondents' usage of AI technology in their clinical orthodontic practice, one multiple-choice item (Q2) examines the potential areas for AI applications in orthodontics based on orthodontists' willingness to adopt it if it proves effective, and one single-choice item (Q3) concerning their interest in AI training and implementation.

- The fifth section, with three items, two Likert-scale questions (Q1 and Q3) and the matrix table questions were included in (Q2), to explore the impact of dental AI on orthodontic practice and assesses how AI influences respondents' clinical decision-making process, diagnosis, treatment planning, and patient experience, as well as their impressions of AI's effect on treatment quality and accuracy in orthodontics.
- Five items were involved in the last section. One multiple-choice item (Q1) encompasses respondents' views on the current challenges and barriers to adopting AI in orthodontics, and the other four are single-choice items to explore the expectations for AI's future evolution in Iraq, its long-term potential, and its transformative impact on orthodontic treatment and workflows.

2.4 Data collection

A web-based anonymous questionnaire was developed and circulated via the Google Forms platform. The scientific research ethics committee at the College of Dentistry, Hawler Medical University (Reference No: HMUD,2425158), on 26/10/2024, approved this study.

Responses were limited to only once per participant to ensure the integrity and neutrality of the research. The questions were structured logically to keep the questionnaire more pertinent and ensure the accuracy in obtaining the responses, as demonstrated in Q3 of Section No. 2. The orthodontists were asked whether they were aware of using AI-powered software programs for diagnosis and treatment planning in orthodontic practice. Based on their response, if they answered 'Yes,' they would be transferred to Q4, Q5, and Q6. If they answered 'No,' they wouldn't be guided to the subsequent three questions. Therefore, depending on the selection made by participants, the next set of questions was either presented or omitted.

An invitation letter and the survey link were sent to the IOS members' orthodontic forum to invite all active members to participate. Three weeks later, the link was resent as a reminder for non-respondents. Additionally, the survey link was sent to the heads of orthodontic departments at universities in Mosul, Duhok, Sulaimani, Najaf, and Karbala.

The first section of the Google form clearly described the purpose of the study, the target survey group, and the appreciation for participation in this research study. Furthermore, participants were notified explicitly that completing the questionnaire is entirely voluntary and would be regarded as granting informed consent for participation.

Participants weren't required to provide a Gmail address or phone number to complete the survey, and no tracking tools were used to ensure respondents' confidentiality. This questionnaire was circulated from January to March 2025.

2.5 Statistical Analysis

Content validity was evaluated based on the CVR of an item and CVI for the overall survey instrument using an Excel workbook "Excel, Microsoft Office LTSC professional plus 2021, Redmond, Washington, USA" to compile and save feedback from both phases of content validation. Face validation was analyzed by computing percent agreement in the same Excel software program and Cohen's kappa statistics using the DATAtab software in a Paid subscription version "DATAtab Team (2025). DATAtab: Online Statistics Calculator. DATAtab e.U. Graz, Austria. URL https://datatab.net." Descriptive statistics were performed using IBM SPSS Statistics version 27.0 (IBM Corp., Armonk, NY, USA) software to categorize the respondents' age groups. Statistical significance was established at a p-value of less than 0.05.

RESULTS

One hundred one active members out of 160 registered orthodontists in the accredited IOS, with higher education credentials in orthodontics, completed the online survey administered from January to March 2025, reflecting a 63% response rate.

Response rate was calculated by dividing the number of survey respondents (101) by the number of contacted and addressed IOS members (160).

Response rate = 101 /160 = 63 %

3.1 Demographic data and professional background

Results illustrated that 101 participants ranged in age from 28 to 67 years, with a mean age of (41.3±7.9). Over one-third were between 38 and 47 years old (46.5%). (53.5%) were females, and (46.5%) were males. The majority of respondents (64.4%) had an MSc, and (35.6%) had a PhD in orthodontics. A large proportion of participating specialists had over ten years of clinical expertise in the orthodontic field. Orthodontic specialists from diverse institutions across Iraq were included in the study sample. Furthermore, the participants in this survey were primarily affiliated with the Ministry of Higher Education and Scientific Research (61.4%); next came those affiliated with the Ministry of Health (36.6%) and mainly based in the northern region of Iraq (48.5%) followed by the central region of Iraq (39.6%). (Table 3.1) summarizes respondents' demographic information and professional background.

Table 3. 1: Demographic data and professional background of the survey participants (n=101).

Characteristics	n (%)
Gender	
Female	54 (53.5%)
Male	47 (46.5%)
Age groups (Years)	
28-37	36 (35.3%)
38-47	47 (46.5%)
48-57	15 (14.9%)
58-67	3 (3%)
Highest academic qualification	
MSc in orthodontics	65 (64.4%)
PhD in orthodontics	36 (35.6%)
Years of clinical experience in orthodontics	
<5 Years	22 (21.8%)
5-10 Years	28 (27.7%)
>10 Years	51 (50.5%)
Institutional information	
Ministry of Health	37 (36.6%)
Ministry of Higher Education and Scientific Research	62 (61.4%)
Others	2 (2%)
Region of residence	
Northern region of Iraq	49 (48.5%)
Central region of Iraq	40 (39.6%)
Southern region of Iraq	6 (5.9%)
Eastern region of Iraq	3 (3%)
Western region of Iraq	3 (3%)

*n=frequency, %=percentage

*Others: refers to orthodontists affiliated with other ministries or not affiliated with any ministry.

3.2 Knowledge and Awareness of AI

As illustrated in (Figure 3.1), professional education (45.5%) and social media (41.6%) were the main sources for learning about AI software programs specifically designed for orthodontics, followed by web browsing (33.7%), scientific journals and books (23.8%), family and colleagues (14.9%), while (11.9%) of participants stated that they had never obtained AI-related information from any source.

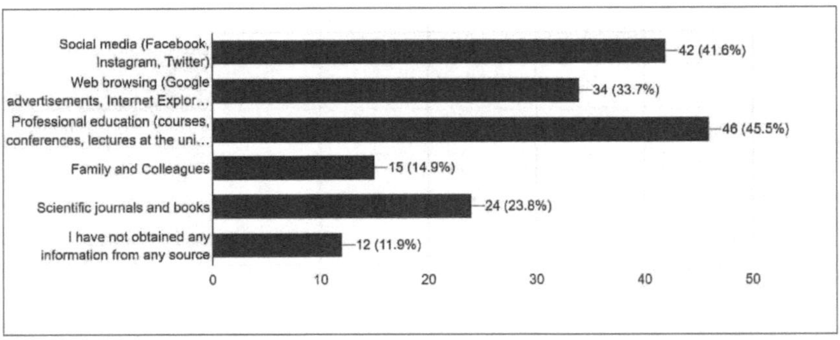

Figure 3. 1: AI Knowledge and awareness reference points for the participants

Among the respondents, 40.6% reported never using any AI orthodontic software. WebCeph was the most commonly used AI software program, with 35.6% of participants indicating its use. Additionally, 21.8% of respondents reported using other AI-based orthodontic software programs. The least commonly used software was NEMOFAB, reported by only (2.0%) of participants. (Figure 3.2).

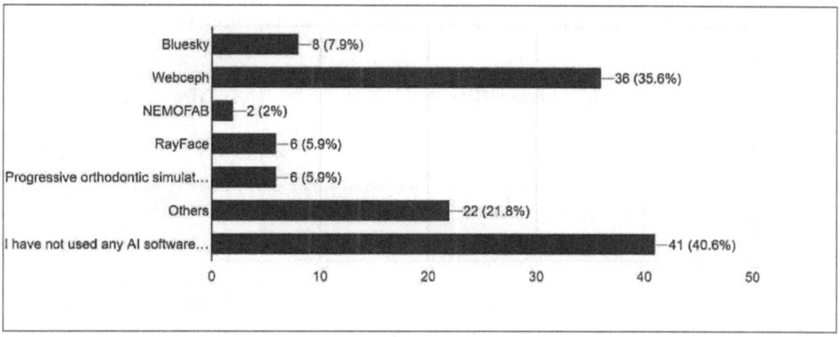

Figure 3. 2: Distribution of AI orthodontic software usage among respondents.

Out of 101 participants, 61.4% reported awareness of using AI-driven software programs for orthodontic diagnosis and treatment planning, while 38.6% indicated they were unaware of such tools.

(Table 3.2) represents a summary of orthodontists' knowledge and awareness of AI regarding (Q4-Q6) in this section. Among (61.4%) of the respondents who stated their awareness of AI-based software programs for diagnosis and treatment planning, (98.4%) were highly aware of the use of AI in digitization and lateral cephalometric analysis, followed by (67.7 %) of them were knowledgeable about AI's role in the preparation and planning for orthognathic surgery and in correcting facial aesthetics. In comparison, only (41.9%) were familiar with using AI-based tools to predict canine impaction, determine the geometry of orthodontic springs to apply force for teeth alignment, and software for selecting the appropriate headgear.

Table 3. 2: Orthodontists' knowledge and awareness of AI regarding responses to (Q4-Q6) in section No. 2 (n=62).

No.	Characteristics	Yes n (%)	No n (%)
Q4	Awareness of AI use in digitization and lateral cephalometric analysis	61 (98.4%)	1 (1.6%)
Q5	Awareness of AI's role in the preparation and planning for orthognathic surgery or in the correction of facial aesthetics	42 (67.7%)	20 (32.3%)
Q6	Familiarity with using AI-assisted tools, such as for the prediction of canine impaction, determining the geometry of orthodontic springs to apply force for teeth alignment, and software for selecting the appropriate headgear	26 (41.9%)	36 (58.1%)

*n=frequency, %=percentage

3.3 Perception about the use of AI in orthodontic practice

A total of 101(52.5%) respondents confirmed the role of AI in saving time for diagnosis and treatment planning in orthodontics. However, (46.5%) expressed a notable level of uncertainty, while only (1.0%) rejected the role of AI in this perspective.

When the surveyed specialists were questioned on whether they had faced differences between artificial intelligence decision-making and their own clinical decision, a significant portion of respondents (79.2%) reported they would trust their own clinical judgments. In contrast, (17.8%) expressed uncertainty in this aspect, while only (3.0%) indicated trust in the AI's decision.

Participating orthodontists expressed diverse perspectives regarding the effectiveness of AI-powered software for diagnosis and treatment planning compared to experienced orthodontists. Interestingly, (49.5%) refused the idea that AI performance surpasses that of professional specialists, (47.5%) indicated uncertainty, and only (3.0%) perceived that AI-powered software might exceed the diagnostic and treatment planning abilities of the specialist orthodontists.

3.4 Attitudes about the use of AI in orthodontics

Concerning the use of AI-powered tools in orthodontic practice, (33.7%) of the surveyed orthodontic specialists reported frequent usage of AI-based tools in their clinical practice. In comparison (32.7%) indicated rare usage, and (30.7%) reported no usage. Only (3.0%) of participants mentioned consistent and regular usage of AI-driven tools in their orthodontic clinical practice.

The survey findings offer profound insights into orthodontists' perspectives on AI integration in orthodontics. Over half of the respondents (61.4%) supported AI applications for clear aligner treatment. Similarly, CBCT and lateral cephalometric analysis with simulation (57.4%) and diagnosis (55.4%) were among the most promising areas for AI implementation in orthodontics. Additionally, (50.5%) of respondents expressed interest in AI applications for patient education and communication. In contrast, biomechanical determination of orthodontic treatment (12.9%) was reported as the least preferred area for AI implementation in orthodontics. (Figure 3.3).

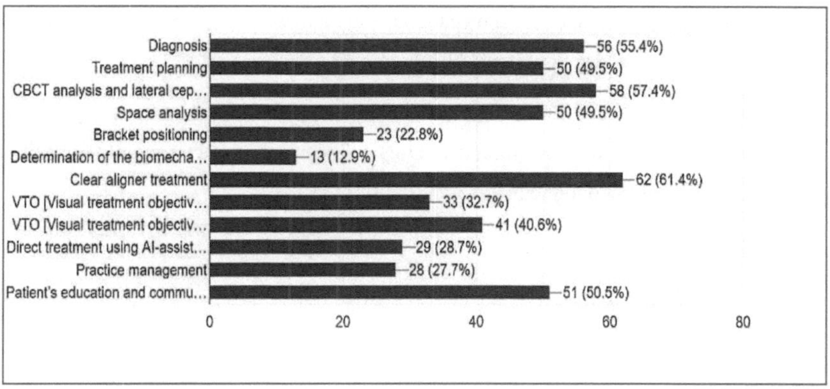

Figure 3. 3: Attitudes toward AI implementation across different orthodontic domains.

Notably, the vast majority of surveyed Iraqi orthodontists (94.1%) expressed a strong desire to undergo formal AI training in orthodontics and incorporate AI-powered tools into their clinical practice. Conversely, only (5.9%) showed no interest in the subject.

3.5 Impact of dental AI in orthodontic practice

The results revealed varying degrees to which AI influences clinical decision-making in orthodontic diagnosis and treatment planning. Of the 101 respondents, 50.5% observed that AI somewhat improved their clinical decision-making capabilities, while 16.8% indicated significant improvement. In contrast, 32.7% reported no impact. Interestingly, none of the participants in the surveyed group reported any adverse impact, suggesting a generally favorable perception of AI among Iraqi orthodontists.

Additionally, the survey examined the influence of dental AI on three fundamental aspects of orthodontic practice: efficiency, accuracy in orthodontic diagnosis and treatment planning, and patient experience, as summarized in (Figure 3.4).

In the context of efficiency, (39.0%) of respondents rated a positive impact, (57.0%) rated neutral, and (5.0%) indicated a negative impact.

Regarding accuracy, (21.0%) of participants observed a positive impact, approximately (72.0%) perceived a neutral impact, and (8.0%) expressed a negative impact.

Finally, concerning the impact of AI on patients' experiences, (39.0%) mentioned a positive influence, (54.0%) rated neutral, and (8.0%) reported a negative effect.

These findings highlighted a neutral perception of dental AI's impact on these key areas of orthodontics. Furthermore, the minimal rating of negative impact supports a positive impression of AI in orthodontic practice in Iraq.

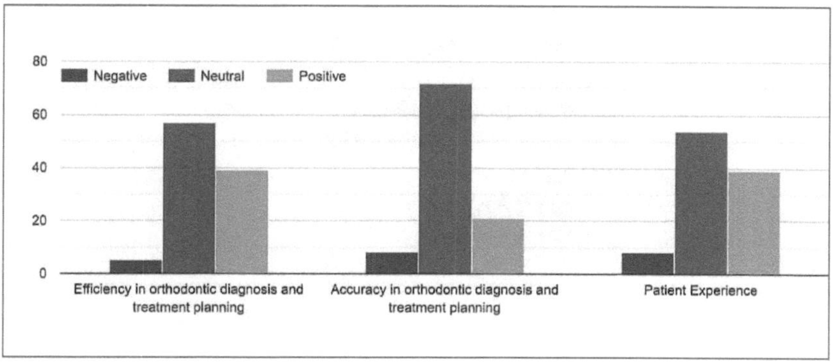

Figure 3. 4: Impact of dental AI on efficiency and accuracy in orthodontic diagnosis and treatment planning as well as patient experience.

Regarding AI's proficiency in improving treatment quality and accuracy in orthodontics, just over half of the surveyed specialists (53.5%) reported agreement, while (8.9%) strongly agreed. However, (2.0%) expressed disagreement, and (7.9%) strongly disagreed. Meanwhile, (27.7%) maintained a neutral perspective.

3.6 The challenges, limitations, and future of AI in orthodontics

This survey study further examined the challenges and concerns associated with adopting AI in orthodontics, as represented in (Figure 3.5). The primary challenge identified was the high cost of creation and design, reported by (68.3%) of respondents. This was followed by a lack of training (61.4%) and concerns regarding accuracy and effectiveness (49.5%). Notably, only (16.8%) of respondents had concerns about data privacy.

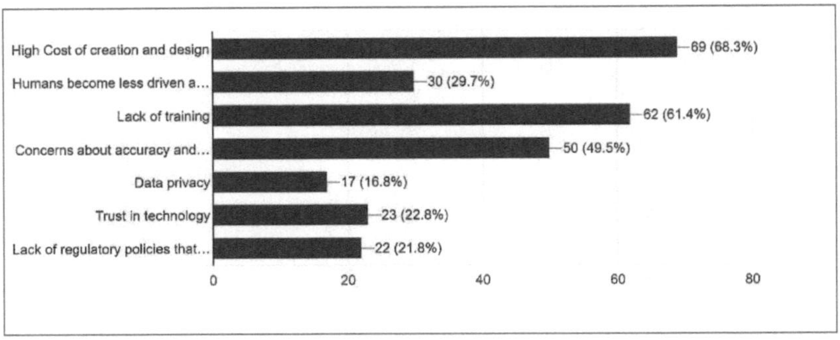

Figure 3. 5: Distribution of challenges for integrating AI in orthodontic practice.

When surveyed participants were asked about the potential of artificial intelligence to take over the role of orthodontists in clinical settings effectively. Over half of the participants (59.4%) strongly rejected the idea, suggesting that AI is not capable of replacing orthodontists. Only a small minority (6.9%) believed that AI could substitute orthodontists in clinical practice. Alternatively, (33.7%) remained uncertain, indicating a 'maybe' response.

Among the participating orthodontists, (45.5%) expressed confidence in using AI-driven programs as a supplementary tool for clinical decision-making in complex cases in the near future. In contrast, (48.5%) of respondents indicated uncertainty, while only (5.9%) entirely rejected this concept.

Concerning the views of Iraqi orthodontic specialists on AI's role in the future of orthodontics, a predominant (60.4%) of respondents anticipated a significant role for AI, reflecting an overall positive outlook. Meanwhile, (37.6%) reported uncertainty, and only (2.0%) expected AI to play no substantial role in the future of orthodontics in Iraq.

Regarding the views of orthodontic specialists in Iraq on integrating AI-related education and training into undergraduate and postgraduate orthodontic programs, a substantial percentage (95.0%) of the 101 surveyed specialists strongly supported the idea. In contrast, only (5.0%) expressed disapproval.

DISCUSSION

4.1 Discussion of the study's objectives and the survey structure

In today's AI-driven world, orthodontics is embracing a revolutionary shift, surpassing the confines of traditional clinical approaches, which makes it essential for orthodontists to stay updated with AI technology and advancements. This study was designed to perform a valid survey to explore the current level of awareness and the extent to which Iraqi orthodontists are implementing AI-driven tools and programs in orthodontic diagnosis, treatment planning, patient management, and monitoring with other possible AI applications and to support orthodontic professionals with a valuable guide to assist in advancing future interdisciplinary research and innovation. Although multiple previous studies (Khanagar et al., 2021c; Seram et al., 2021; Aboalshamat, 2022; Murali et al., 2023; Lin et al., 2023; Jeong et al., 2024; Kharroubi et al., 2024; Bhanotia et al., 2024; Hegde et al., 2025) have assessed dental professionals' and students' knowledge and attitudes toward AI applications. The evaluation of specialists' adoption in orthodontics is particularly limited within the Iraqi context and more broadly across the MENA countries.

During the survey's validation process, three items were rated as essential by only five experts. They were considered significant and retained by the researchers based on their relevance and important applicability. These questions are: -

- Question No. 2 in section No. 2, which included the question (Which AI orthodontic software have you used?) was incorporated to assess the firsthand experience of Iraqi orthodontists with AI-powered orthodontic software, and this will provide insights into familiarity, accessibility, and the level of practical integration of AI in the clinical settings. Moreover, it helps to explore whether direct experience with AI tools influences orthodontists' perception and willingness to incorporate AI into their clinical workflows. Among the options chosen to be included was the Webceph software because it is a well-known AI software used for diagnosis and cephalometric analysis, and is available in both free and affordable paid subscription options. A large percentage of specialists were expected to be familiar with it. However, despite being the most commonly used AI software program among participants, only 35.6% of the 101 respondents reported familiarity with its usage.

The Bluesky program was recommended for inclusion by a member of the expert panel for content validation who was familiar with its functionalities. At the time of survey instrument development, RayFace was a newly introduced AI-powered facial scanner in the country. Similarly, the progressive orthodontic app represented an innovative, groundbreaking revolution in orthodontics; therefore, there was a consensus to include these two programs in the multiple-choice options. NEMOFAB is an AI-driven digital platform offering comprehensive analysis of facial, airway, and bite (FAB) characteristics correction as well as planning for orthognathic surgery. Notably, it is also available at an affordable subscription price.

Although more than half of orthodontists (61.4%) expressed positive awareness of using AI-powered software programs for diagnosis and treatment planning, A significant (40.6%) of respondents reported that they had never used any AI-driven orthodontic software, underscoring a notable gap in AI adoption in clinical orthodontic practice. This may result from several challenges, including financial constraints, unfamiliarity with the technology, doubts about its efficiency and accuracy, and a lack of well-organized workshops and educational webinars in this field in the country.

- Question No. 3 in section No. 4 (Would you be interested in receiving formal training on AI in orthodontics and integrating AI-based tools into your practice?) aimed to examine whether specialists' perceptions of AI in orthodontic practice correlate with their willingness to pursue AI training for further knowledge enhancement.
- Question No. 2 in section No. 6 (Do you believe artificial intelligence could substitute orthodontists in clinical practice?) was included to assess whether there is concern about job replacement by AI-driven technologies. It provides insights into whether orthodontists view AI as a supportive tool that enhances their work or as a potential competitor that could threaten their professional role in clinical practice.

4.2 Discussion and comparison of the study's main and different results

The lowest percentage of participants in this survey came from the southern, eastern, and western regions of Iraq. This is attributed to the shortage of orthodontic specialists in these regions, unlike in the northern and central areas of the country.

The awareness of AI applications in digitization and lateral cephalometric analysis was notably high among the participants, exceeding their awareness of AI's role in orthognathic surgery, facial aesthetic corrections, and other specialized orthodontic applications. In particular, knowledge and familiarity with AI's potential in predicting canine impaction and in biomechanical domains, such as optimizing the geometry of orthodontic springs for precise force application and selecting appropriate headgear appliances, were comparatively low.

Furthermore, AI-driven cephalometric analysis and simulation were among the most well-accepted applications, with participants expressing strong positive attitudes toward their integration into clinical practice. This can be explained by:

- Numerous AI-driven platforms for cephalometric digitization and analysis are currently available. Some are freely accessible, while others are offered at reasonable prices, which has enhanced their widespread adoption and utilization in orthodontic practice.
- An extensive volume of evidence-based studies supporting the reliability of various AI-driven software products in cephalometric digitization and analysis has played a key role in fostering user trust in these tools' applications. In a review by (Surendran et al., 2024) Stated that AI's most impactful role in orthodontics is its exceptional accuracy in detecting landmarks on lateral cephalograms, standing out as a leading application. (Katyal and Balakrishnan, 2022) assessed the accuracy of three approaches for cephalometric analysis, including manual tracing, digital-based FACAD, and AI-driven Webceph. The Webceph proved efficient, reliable, and convenient compared to the other two methods. Moreover, research by (Chuchra et al., 2024) compared the accuracy of three programs, OneCeph, NemoCeph, and Webceph, with traditional manual tracing and concluded that these software programs are credible and dependable.

The limited awareness of AI's role in orthognathic surgery and biomechanical simulation indicates a need for more training, exposure, and evidence-based validation to encourage specialists and improve AI implementation in these areas.

Our study demonstrated that while more than half of the participants believed that AI could efficiently boost treatment accuracy in orthodontics, streamline clinical workflows, and reduce diagnosis and treatment planning time. Furthermore, the overwhelming majority of orthodontists are willing to undergo formal training on AI in orthodontics and to integrate it into clinical practice. There were doubts about AI decisions, where the significant majority (more than three-quarters) indicated they would depend on their own clinical judgments if conflicts were encountered between their decisions and those made by AI. Moreover, nearly half of the participants rejected the idea that AI's effectiveness surpasses that of professional orthodontists, while more than a third remained uncertain, possibly due to factors like unfamiliarity with AI's decision-making process or perceived limitations in reliability.

Orthodontics is a highly proficient specialty. In a narrative review by (Tahir et al., 2024) It has been emphasized that adopting AI does not change the essential role of orthodontists, who depend on their in-depth knowledge, extensive training, and experience to make accurate diagnoses and formulate optimal treatment strategies. Ethics must remain a priority, as devices and robots cannot provide the compassion and emotional intelligence that human physicians have.(Rokaya et al., 2024).

The apprehension could further be justified by AI's limited ability and inherent challenges in adapting to the complexities of clinical decision-making. Effective healthcare relies on a strong physician-patient relationship marked by open and honest communication based on trust and compassion, which is essential for successful medical care. However, the implementation of AI challenges the conventional physician-patient collaboration, which centres on the clinician's sophisticated and multifaceted comprehension of the patient's state of wellness and overall history, and might fail to recognize the critical psychological, mental, and cultural variables that are essential to the individual's health and comfort.(Mennella et al., 2024)

This is why participants in this survey were more inclined to trust their own clinical judgment. They appreciated the contextual and personalized understanding that comes with human interaction, a quality that AI can never fully and truly replicate.

Regarding the field of biomechanics, orthodontists displayed the least awareness, familiarity, and support for AI integration. This contrasts sharply with their strong positive attitudes toward AI adoption in clear aligner treatment. This could be attributed to the perception that biomechanics is a vital field in orthodontics that relies heavily on orthodontists' professional judgment, skills, or hands-on expertise. This aspect may lie beyond the capabilities of AI. The relatively limited availability of supportive and specialized programs in biomechanics, combined with a lack of marketing initiatives, webinars, or workshops aimed at promoting AI tools in this field, is especially apparent when compared to other areas, such as AI adoption in clear aligners, where such resources are more prevalent.

This is exemplified by the widespread availability of various clear aligner providers, the strong marketing strategies for different types of aligners, and the numerous workshops, webinars, and lectures held nearly continuously worldwide, particularly the superior, widely recognized Invisalign® technique (Weir, 2017).In addition to the extensive research demonstrating the effectiveness of clear aligners in treating various case scenarios, providing evidence-based validation for specialists has also boosted user confidence in these tools.

It is worth mentioning that many research has demonstrated the efficiency of applying intelligent technology in specific domains of biomechanics, particularly the proven results and efficiency achieved by an ANN-based AI system designed by (Kazem et al., 2010) for evaluating the optimal force of the " T-retraction spring". Given the rapid advancements in research and development in this field, we can expect the creation of more comprehensive AI products that address every aspect of orthodontics.

Despite the significant potential of AI, its daily application in dental practice remains limited. It is still viewed as being in its early stages and has yet to fully realize its capabilities or achieve comprehensive integration (Mengi et al., 2024). This may explain why just 3.0% of participants consistently incorporate AI into their practice, while 33.7%

use it frequently. Furthermore, more than half of the participants described the impact of AI on the efficiency and accuracy of orthodontic diagnosis, treatment planning, and patient experience as 'neutral.' Additionally, only half of the participants perceived a slight improvement in their clinical decision-making, with a small minority reporting a significant improvement. Another possible justification is the reported gap in the published research regarding security and confidentiality concerns, algorithm honesty, and the need for thorough evaluation and standardization procedures (Shafi et al., 2024). Furthermore, the cost issues associated with implementing AI technology may present challenges for certain procedures. Therefore, there is an urgent need for ongoing education to remain updated with technological innovations to overcome significant obstacles (Tahir et al., 2024).

This survey revealed that the majority of participants believed orthodontists could never be replaced by AI, with only 6.9% in agreement. Meanwhile, more than one-third expressed confidence in relying on AI as a secondary tool for judgment in challenging cases, and 5.9% rejected this concept. This can be interpreted as AI generally being perceived as a collaborator, supporter, and complementary tool in orthodontic decision-making.

In a narrative review by (Mennella et al., 2024) It was emphasized that AI must be considered exclusively a resource to assist clinicians in their clinical decision-making process, which must always be managed and controlled by human physicians. The programmed intellectual support mechanism in medical diagnosis and treatment could never be compared with self-regulating decisions. AI demonstrated several inaccuracies in evaluation and assessment. Therefore, a qualified clinician must conduct the final inspection to prevent these kinds of mistakes (Rokaya et al., 2024).

4.3 Discussion and comparison with other different Surveys' results

No up-to-date studies have been published regarding the assessment of perception and application of dental artificial intelligence that exclusively targeted orthodontic specialists.

The latest published surveys in orthodontic communities in other regions worldwide addressed the following:

- "Knowledge, experience, and attitudes on AI-assisted cephalometric analysis by orthodontists and orthodontic students". (Lin et al., 2023)
- "A questionnaire study regarding knowledge, attitude, and usage of AI and ML by the orthodontic fraternity of Northern India".(Mengi et al., 2024)
- "Training, use, and modifications related to artificial intelligence in postgraduate orthodontic programs in North America".(Hanenkrath et al., 2025)
- "Knowledge, attitude, and perception regarding the role of AI in the orthodontic field by orthodontists and orthodontic students".(Gupta et al., 2025)

Regarding the sources of AI knowledge and awareness, the primary source was professional education. This finding is in accordance with those of other surveys (Lin et al., 2023; Gupta et al., 2025), but in contrast to a study conducted by (Mengi et al., 2024), where the major sources were web browsing and social media.

61.4% of specialists participating in this study were aware of AI use for diagnosis and treatment planning. Regarding the treatment planning, this observation aligns with the results obtained by (Gupta et al., 2025) where 61% of the orthodontic faculty members agreed that AI can be used for treatment planning.

Our results are in reasonable proximity to those reported in a survey by (Gupta et al., 2025). Overall, their findings indicate a general expectation that AI will play a significant role and have a promising future in orthodontic practice. Lateral cephalometric analysis was among the well-recognized AI applications with notable practitioner awareness. AI-assisted cephalometric software, according to (Lin et al., 2023), has the potential to replace manual and semiautomated methods and make cephalometric analysis more manageable and more accessible for clinicians. In a scoping review by (Mohammad-Rahimi et al., 2021), cephalometric digitization and analysis were ranked among the most favorable and guaranteed AI applications.

In contrast to the findings reported by (Gupta et al., 2025) Our survey results revealed differing perspectives among Iraqi orthodontists in several key areas. The following points highlight where our findings diverge from theirs:

- While Gupta et al.'s research reported that only 16.0 % of their participants had more than ten years of clinical experience in orthodontics, our study indicated that half of the participating orthodontists possessed over ten years of clinical experience. This can be justified by the fact that the current study explored knowledge and attitudes among only specialists, unlike Gupta et al.'s, which included orthodontists and orthodontic residents.
- Unlike Gupta et al.'s participants, in whom only (63.33%) of the faculty orthodontic members expressed a willingness to attend professional training, the results of our study demonstrated the interest of a predominant portion (94.1 %) of orthodontists in receiving formal training and integrating AI-powered tools into their clinical practice.
- Whereas Gupta et al.'s survey revealed that 44.67 % of orthodontists agreed that AI has better diagnostic ability than experienced orthodontists, the present study indicated that only a small minority (3.0 %) perceived that the performance of AI-driven tools might exceed that of a professional orthodontist.

In addition to differing from Gupta et al., the outcomes of the current survey also stand in contrast to those conducted by (Mengi et al., 2024) in the following two aspects :

- Mengi et al. reported that the vast majority (90.0%) indicated that the incorporation of AI into CBCT analysis is an important addition to the diagnosis and treatment plan. On the contrary, over half of the participants in this study (57.4%) demonstrated that the integration of AI in CBCT analysis is promising.
- While 84.0% of Mengi et al. participants agreed that AI could enhance the performance and quality of orthodontic care, the present study demonstrated that over half of the participants (53.5%) concurred that AI could improve the quality and accuracy of orthodontic treatment.

41.0 % of the participants in this survey were aware of AI's role in preparing and planning orthognathic surgery. These results did not align with the study conducted by (Gupta et al., 2025), where 74.0 % of faculty members endorsed the use of AI in 3D planning for orthognathic surgery, nor the study by (Mengi et al., 2024) , in which 86.0 % of respondents agreed that AI could assist in clinical judgment for orthognathic surgery.

Half of the participants in this study perceived that AI could assist in saving time and streamlining clinical processes workflow. In a survey by (Lin et al., 2023), It was indicated that the most significant benefit of utilizing AI methods for cephalometric analysis was the time savings, which served as the primary incentive for most to embrace this approach.

An impressive percentage of participants in this survey (95.0%) strongly recommended incorporating AI training in undergraduate and postgraduate programs curricula. Concerning postgraduate training, a lower percentage was observed in the findings of the survey by (Gupta et al., 2025), where 75.0 % of orthodontists recommended AI integration in postgraduate training. In a most recent study by (Hanenkrath et al., 2025), it was reported that only half of the North American postgraduate orthodontic programs have implemented or are planning to implement AI in certain aspects, and 87.8% indicated that they had not incorporated any seminar or training into their programs to train the orthodontic residents.

The biggest and primary challenge for adopting AI in orthodontics, as reported by the surveyed participants, was the high cost of creation and design (68.3%). This is opposed to the findings from the survey by (Gupta et al., 2025), in which orthodontists reported that the main barrier to adopting AI in orthodontics was a lack of technical knowledge (94.67%).Additionally, another survey by (Mengi et al., 2024), less human interaction with the patient was the major concern.

This survey indicated that more than three-quarters of specialists chose to depend on their clinical decisions if conflicts are encountered with AI's decisions. This finding reflects the findings of a recent study by (Mengi et al., 2024).

4.4 Key strengths of the current study

- This research stands as the first and uniquely original study of its kind conducted in Iraq regarding the types and procedures of validation, subsequently considering its defined scope to investigate specialist orthodontists' knowledge and inspect their perceptions and attitudes toward the application of dental AI-driven tools and software into their clinical practice. The survey contents were validated using Lawshe's method. Despite the ease of calculating Lawshe's CVR, its interpretation can be complex as its scores lie between -1.0 and +1.0; a CVR of zero indicates that half of the experts considered an item relevant, and such items are often excluded, as zero falls below the acceptable threshold.(Polit et al., 2007)
- Moreover, this survey instrument was validated by six academics and expert specialists in orthodontics from various geographical locations and four prestigious universities across Iraq for content validation, as well as by two additional expert panels for face validation. The panel of experts was highly experienced and well-qualified to assess the field under study. The criteria for selecting the expert panel, the comprehensive information they received regarding the design of the questionnaire, the content validation procedures, and the format of the invitation letter were all consistent with the guidelines authored by (Grant and Davis, 1997).In conclusion, this survey instrument had (CVI=0.96), which reflects excellent content validity as recommended by (Waltz et al., 2005) , and (k=0.72), which falls within the good strength level of Cohen's kappa statistics of 0.61 and more, as recommended by (Altman, 1999).
- The target survey group: This survey specifically targeted orthodontic specialists who possess advanced training and a comprehensive understanding of orthodontic principles. Since specialists are at the forefront of integrating new technologies through research, training, or direct patient care, they represent the most qualified group to assess perceptions, attitudes, and clinical applications of AI in orthodontics. Understanding their views helps predict AI's potential influence on clinical orthodontic practice, ensuring that responses are informed by professional experience and knowledge rather than general opinions. This approach leads to more reliable and meaningful findings, thereby strengthening the research's validity by capturing experts' perspectives on AI in the orthodontic field in Iraq.

- Furthermore, this survey achieved a 63% response rate, significantly exceeding the 44.0% threshold recommended for online surveys as reported in a meta-analysis by (Wu et al., 2022).This high response rate strengthens the validity, generalizability, and robustness of the survey findings. Moreover, this active participation rate underscores the significance of the research topic and further reinforces the study's clinical and academic relevance.

4.5 Limitations of the current research

Considering the scope of this research, it is essential to address the following limitations:

- Sample size-related bias can be attributed to two main reasons:
  - ➢ Not all orthodontic specialists in Iraq are registered with the Iraqi Orthodontic Society.
  - ➢ The sample may not fully represent the wider population, as the principle under investigation is likely to be more familiar and easily understood by younger individuals than by older ones.
- Voluntary self-preference bias, which can be explained by two key factors :
  - ➢ Given the voluntary nature of the response, election bias is inevitable, as respondents were likely those with a preexisting interest in AI.
  - ➢ Self-reported response bias might restrict the generalizability of our findings, particularly for individuals who have not used AI in orthodontics, possess inadequate knowledge, or have had negative experiences with AI technology. Additionally, the condition and the setting in which the survey was administered could have impacted the responses, introducing bias. This may have, in turn, compromised the accuracy of the data recorded by the respondents, possibly due to rushing or insufficient attention paid to the questions.

CONCLUSIONS AND RECOMMENDATIONS

5.1 Conclusions

The survey study assessed orthodontic specialists' perceptions and adoption of dental AI to understand its current implementation level in Iraq's orthodontic practice. The following conclusions were drawn: -.

- Overall, there was a good level of awareness and knowledge about AI's role in diagnosis and treatment planning, with notable openness and a strong willingness among specialists to participate in AI-related training and incorporate it into their professional routines.
- Despite this, a clear gap exists in the actual implementation of AI within orthodontic practice.
- AI is regarded as a complementary and augmentative tool rather than a replacement for experienced professionals.
- The future of artificial intelligence in orthodontics is viewed positively, and there is widespread consensus on the significance of its integration into undergraduate and postgraduate programs.
- The research underscores the need for further education, training, evidence-based validation, and the development of more AI-powered tools targeting different areas of orthodontics, especially biomechanics.
- Orthodontists should be encouraged to adopt AI as a supportive tool while prioritizing patient well-being in clinical decision-making.

5.2 Recommendations

Drawing from the conclusions of this study, the following recommendations are proposed to improve the current landscape of AI integration in orthodontics and to address the key issues identified during the research:

- Expanding educational, training, and awareness initiatives, along with well-structured workshops and webinars, is crucial to familiarize professionals with the benefits and practical application of AI-powered programs in orthodontics. Well-designed educational programs, seminars, and workshops could support wider adoption.
- Raising awareness and improving education on AI integration in orthodontic biomechanics, increasing research efforts, and developing advanced AI-based models tailored to this field are essential steps towards innovation in orthodontic practice. These efforts aim to bridge the trust gap and foster confidence among orthodontists.
- Promote cooperation between orthodontists and AI programmers to fix challenges and incorporate professional human skills into AI tasks.
- It would be highly beneficial to carry out longitudinal studies to explore the impact of incorporating AI into undergraduate and postgraduate orthodontic curricula and assess the effectiveness of various educational and training approaches.
- Conducting research to examine the long-term effects of AI applications in orthodontics, including patient education and monitoring, accuracy of diagnosis, formulated clinical decisions, and care effectiveness, will enhance our understanding of how AI technologies shape orthodontic clinical practice and provide evidence-based foundations that support AI's validity.
- To further enhance the understanding of dental AI application in orthodontic practice in Iraq, the following topics are proposed for future questionnaire research:

➢ Knowledge, awareness, and application of dental AI among higher education orthodontic candidates in Iraq. The findings could support evidence-based curriculum enhancement, development, and AI integration in orthodontic education.

- Perceptions, attitudes, and clinical and academic training related to employing dental AI in higher education orthodontic programs in Iraqi universities. This would help identify gaps and opportunities for improvement in AI-related orthodontic training and develop AI-integrated curricula to enhance orthodontic education.
- Conducting a similar study that includes both general practitioners and specialists, and analyzing the differences between the two groups in terms of their knowledge, perception, and attitudes towards implementing dental AI in orthodontic practice. This would offer a broader understanding of how AI is perceived and used across various levels of dental expertise.

REFERENCES

Abdelkarim A, Jerrold L (2017). Orthodontic chart documentation. Am J Orthod Dentofacial Orthop;152 (1):126–30.

Aboalshamat KT (2022). Perception and Utilization of Artificial Intelligence (AI) among Dental Professionals in Saudi Arabia. Open Dent J; 16(1):e187421062208110.

Abutayyem H, Asim Alsalam AA, Iqbal RM, Alkhabuli J, El-Din Mohamed SK (2019). Robotic Use in Orthodontics: Literature Review. Oral Health Dent Sci; 3(3):16-18.

Ackerman MB (2003). The myth of Janus: orthodontic progress faces orthodontic history. Am J Orthod Dentofacial Orthop; 123(6):594–6.

Agrawal P, Nikhade P (2022). Artificial Intelligence in Dentistry: Past, Present, and Future. Cureus; 14 (7):e27405.

Akçam MO, Takada K (2002). Fuzzy modelling for selecting headgear types. Eur J Orthod; 24(1):99–106.

Akkaya N, Ünsal G, Orhan K, editors (2023). Understanding of AI in Dental Field with Technical Aspects. Artif. Intell. Dent., Cham: Springer International Publishing; [cited 2025 Mar 1]. p. 9–29. Available from: https://link.springer.com/10.1007/978-3-031-43827-1.

Al Mortadi N, Eggbeer D, Lewis J, Williams RJ (2012). CAD/CAM/AM applications in the manufacture of dental appliances. Am J Orthod Dentofacial Orthop; 142(5):727–33.

Albalawi F, Alamoud KA (2022). Trends and Application of Artificial Intelligence Technology in Orthodontic Diagnosis and Treatment Planning—A Review. Appl Sci; 12(22):11864.

Aldrees AM (2016). Do customized orthodontic appliances and vibration devices provide more efficient treatment than conventional methods? Korean J Orthod; 46(3):180.

Alkhal HA, Wong RWK, Rabie ABM (2008). Correlation between Chronological Age, Cervical Vertebral Maturation and Fishman's Skeletal Maturity Indicators in Southern Chinese. Angle Orthod; 78(4):591–6.

Al-Moghrabi D, Barber S, Fleming PS (2021). Removable retention: enhancing adherence and the remit of shared decision-making. Br Dent J; 230(11):765–9.

Al-Naseri YAY (2017). A randomised clinical trial of the effectiveness of orthodontic treatment between the 0.018-inch and the 0.022-inch slot conventional ligation bracket systems. PhD Thesis. University of Dundee. United Kingdom.

Alowais SA, Alghamdi SS, Alsuhebany N, Alqahtani T, Alshaya AI, Almohareb SN, et al (2023). Revolutionizing healthcare: the role of artificial intelligence in clinical practice. BMC Med Educ; 23(1):689.

Altman DG (1999). Practical statistics for medical research. 1st ed. Boca Raton, Fla: Chapman & Hall/CRC. P.403-9.

Arik SÖ, Ibragimov B, Xing L (2017). Fully automated quantitative cephalometry using convolutional neural networks. J Med Imaging; 4(1):014501.

Asiri SN, Tadlock LP, Schneiderman E, Buschang PH (2020). Applications of artificial intelligence and machine learning in orthodontics. APOS Trends Orthod; 10(1):17–24.

Ayad N, Schwendicke F, Krois J, van den Bosch S, Bergé S, Bohner L, et al (2023). Patients' perspectives on the use of artificial intelligence in dentistry: a regional survey. Head Face Med; 19(1):23.

Bahaa K, Noor G, Yousif Y (2011). The artificial intelligence approach for diagnosis, treatment and modelling in orthodontic. Princ Contemp Orthod. 1st ed. Iraq: Baghdad: 451–92.

Bayrakdar IS, Orhan K, Jagtap R, editors (2023). Artificial Intelligence in Dental Education. Artif. Intell. Dent., Cham: Springer International Publishing; [cited 2025 Apr 12]. p. 223–234. Available from: https://link.springer.com/10.1007/978-3-031-43827-1.

Beglin FM, Firestone AR, Vig KWL, Beck FM, Kuthy RA, Wade D (2001). A comparison of the reliability and validity of 3 occlusal indexes of orthodontic treatment need. Am J Orthod Dentofacial Orthop; 120(3):240–6.

Bengel W (2000). Digital photography in the dental practice--an overview (II). Int J Comput Dent;3(2):121–32.

Bhanotia D, Alam ST, Trehan M, Rai D, Rai A (2024). Assessing the AI Acumen: A study on the knowledge, attitude and behaviour of dental students towards artificial intelligence. J Contemp Orthod; 8(3):290–3.

Bichu YM, Zou B, Chaudhari PK, Adel SM, Vaiid N (2025). Artificial Intelligence Applications in Orthodontics. In: Schwendicke F, Chaudhari PK, Dhingra K, Uribe SE, Hamdan M, editors. Artif. Intell. Oral Health Care, Cham: Springer Nature Switzerland; [cited 2025 Apr 10]. p. 81–97. Available from: https://link.springer.com/10.1007/978-3-031-84047-0_6.

Broadbent BH (1931). A new X-ray technique and its application to orthodontia. Angle Orthod; 1(2):45–66.

Butul B, Sharab L (2024). Obstacles to Innovation: A Peek into Artificial Intelligence in the Field of Orthodontics – A Literature Review. Saudi Dent J; 36(6):830–4.

Carmines E, Zeller R (1979). Reliability and Validity Assessment. 2455 Teller Road, Thousand Oaks California 91320 United States of America: SAGE Publications, Inc; [cited 2025 Feb 22]. Available from: https://methods.sagepub.com/book/reliability-and-validity-assessment.

Carrillo-Perez F, Pecho OE, Morales JC, Paravina RD, Della Bona A, Ghinea R, et al (2022). Applications of artificial intelligence in dentistry: A comprehensive review. J Esthet Restor Dent; 34(1):259–80.

Caruso Silvia, Caruso Sara, Pellegrino M, Skafi R, Nota A, Tecco S (2021). A Knowledge-Based Algorithm for Automatic Monitoring of Orthodontic Treatment: The Dental Monitoring System. Two Cases. Sensors; 21(5):1856.

Chandrashekar G, AlQarni S, Bumann EE, Lee Y (2022). Collaborative deep learning model for tooth segmentation and identification using panoramic radiographs. Comput Biol Med; 148(C):105829.

Chen S, Wang L, Li G, Wu T-H, Diachina S, Tejera B, et al (2020). Machine Learning in Orthodontics: *Introducing a 3d Auto-segmentation and Auto-landmark Finder of Cbct Images To Assess Maxillary Constriction in Unilateral Impacted Canine patients*. Angle Orthod; 90(1):77–84.

Chuchra A, Gupta K, Arora R, Bindra S, Hingad N, Babbar A (2024). Digital Cephalometric Analysis: Unveiling the Role and Reliability of Semi-automated OneCeph, Artificial Intelligence-Powered WebCeph Mobile App, and Semi-automated Computer-Aided NemoCeph Software in Orthodontic Practice. Cureus; 16(1):e72948

Claman L, Patton D, Rashid R (1990). Standardized portrait photography for dental patients. Am J Orthod Dentofacial Orthop; 98(3):197–205.

Cohen J (1960). A Coefficient of Agreement for Nominal Scales. Educ Psychol Meas; 20(1):37–46.

Cole D, Bencharit S, Carrico CK, Arias A, Tüfekçi E (2019). Evaluation of fit for 3D-printed retainers compared with thermoform retainers. Am J Orthod Dentofacial Orthop; 155(4):592–9.

Croquet B, Matthews H, Mertens J, Fan Y, Nauwelaers N, Mahdi S, et al (2021). Automated landmarking for palatal shape analysis using geometric deep learning. Orthod Craniofac Res;24(S2):144–52.

Cruciger O, Schildhauer TA, Meindl RC, Tegenthoff M, Schwenkreis P, Citak M, et al (2016). Impact of locomotion training with a neurologic controlled hybrid assistive limb (HAL) exoskeleton on neuropathic pain and health related quality of life (HRQoL) in chronic SCI: a case study*. Disabil Rehabil Assist Technol; 11(6):529–34.

Dashti M, Ghasemi S, Khurshid Z (2024a). Integrating Artificial Intelligence in Dental Education: An Urgent Call for Dedicated Postgraduate Programs. Int Dent J; 74(6):1466–8.

Dashti M, Londono J, Ghasemi S, Khurshid Z, Khosraviani F, Moghaddasi N, et al (2024b). Attitudes, knowledge, and perceptions of dentists and dental students toward artificial intelligence: a systematic review. J Taibah Univ Med Sci; 19(2):327–37.

Davenport T, Kalakota R (2019). The potential for artificial intelligence in healthcare. Future Healthc J; 6(2):94–8.

Davis LL (1992). Instrument review: Getting the most from a panel of experts. Appl Nurs Res; 5(4):194–7.

DeVellis RF (1991). Scale development: Theory and applications. 1st ed. Thousand Oaks, CA, US: Sage Publications, Inc. P. 121.

DeVon HA, Block ME, Moyle-Wright P, Ernst DM, Hayden SJ, Lazzara DJ, et al (2007). A Psychometric Toolbox for Testing Validity and Reliability. J Nurs Scholarsh; 39(2):155–64.

Dhopte A, Bagde H (2023). Smart Smile: Revolutionizing Dentistry With Artificial Intelligence. Cureus; 15(6):e41227

Díaz Ó, Dalton JAR, Giraldo J (2019). Artificial Intelligence: A Novel Approach for Drug Discovery. Trends Pharmacol Sci; 40(8):550–1.

Dietrich CA, Ender A, Baumgartner S, Mehl A (2017). A validation study of reconstructed rapid prototyping models produced by two technologies. Angle Orthod; 87(5):782–7.

DiFranco DE, Cham T-J, Rehg JM (2001). Reconstruction of 3D figure motion from 2D correspondences. Proc. 2001 IEEE Comput. Soc. Conf. Comput. Vis. Pattern Recognit. CVPR 2001, vol. 1, IEEE; 2001[cited 2025 Jan 10]. p. I–I. Available from: https://ieeexplore.ieee.org/abstract/document/990491/.

Ding H, Wu J, Zhao W, Matinlinna JP, Burrow MF, Tsoi JK. (2023) Artificial intelligence in dentistry—A review. Front Dent Med; 4:1085251

Distler V, Lallemand C, Koenig V (2020). How Acceptable Is This? How User Experience Factors Can Broaden our Understanding of The Acceptance of Privacy Trade-offs. Comput Hum Behav; 106:106227.

Dolce C, Mansour DA, McGorray SP, Wheeler TT (2012). Intrarater agreement about the etiology of Class II malocclusion and treatment approach. Am J Orthod Dentofacial Orthop; 141(1):17–23.

Elangovan N, Sundaravel E (2021). Method of preparing a document for survey instrument validation by experts. MethodsX; 8:101326.

Etemad L, Wu T-H, Heiner P, Liu J, Lee S, Chao W-L, et al (2021). Machine learning from clinical data sets of a contemporary decision for orthodontic tooth extraction. Orthod Craniofac Res; 24(S2):193–200.

Ezhov M, Gusarev M, Golitsyna M, Yates JM, Kushnerev E, Tamimi D, et al (2021). Clinically applicable artificial intelligence system for dental diagnosis with CBCT. Sci Rep; 11(1):15006.

Faber J, Faber C, Faber P (2019). Artificial intelligence in orthodontics. APOS Trends Orthod; 9(4):201–5.

Fatima A, Shafi I, Afzal H, Díez IDLT, Lourdes DR-SM, Breñosa J, et al (2022). Advancements in Dentistry with Artificial Intelligence: Current Clinical Applications and Future Perspectives. Healthc Basel Switz; 10:2188.

Fawaz P, Sayegh PE, Vannet BV (2023). What is the current state of artificial intelligence applications in dentistry and orthodontics? J Stomatol Oral Maxillofac Surg; 124(5):101524.

Franco de Sá Gomes C, Libdy MR, Normando D (2019). Scan time, reliability and accuracy of craniofacial measurements using a 3D light scanner. J Oral Biol Craniofacial Res; 9(4):331–5.

Gable RK, Wolf MB (1993). Instrument Development in the Affective Domain. 2nd ed.Dordrecht: Springer Netherlands; [cited 2025 Feb 22]. Available from: http://link.springer.com/10.1007/978-94-011-1400-4.

Gerke S, Minssen T, Cohen G (2020). Chapter 12 - Ethical and legal challenges of artificial intelligence-driven healthcare. In: Bohr A, Memarzadeh K, editors. Artif. Intell. Healthc., Academic Press;[cited 2025 Apr 11]. p. 295–336. Available from: https://www.sciencedirect.com/science/article/pii/B9780128184387000125.

Gianfrancesco MA, Tamang S, Yazdany J, Schmajuk G (2018). Potential Biases in Machine Learning Algorithms Using Electronic Health Record Data. JAMA Intern Med; 178(11):1544–7.

Gilbert GE, Prion S (2016). Making Sense of Methods and Measurement: Lawshe's Content Validity Index. Clin Simul Nurs; 12(12):530–1.

Goh GD, Lee JM, Goh GL, Huang X, Lee S, Yeong WY (2023). Machine Learning for Bioelectronics on Wearable and Implantable Devices: Challenges and Potential. Tissue Eng Part A; 29(1-2):20–46.

Grant JS, Davis LL (1997). Selection and use of content experts for instrument development. Res Nurs Health; 20(3):269–74.

Grant JS, Kinney MR (1992). Using the Delphi Technique to Examine the Content Validity of Nursing Diagnoses. Int J Nurs Terminol Classif; 3(1):12–22.

Gupta S, Verma S, Chauhan AK, Roy MS, Rajkumari W, Sahgal C (2025). Knowledge, attitude, and perception of orthodontic students, and orthodontists regarding role of artificial intelligence in field of orthodontics—An online cross-sectional survey. J World Fed Orthod; 14(1):3–11.

Hamet P, Tremblay J (2017). Artificial intelligence in medicine. Metabolism; 69S:S36–40.

Han UK, Vig KWL, Weintraub JA, Vig PS, Kowalski CJ (1991). Consistency of orthodontic treatment decisions relative to diagnostic records. Am J Orthod Dentofacial Orthop; 100(3):212–9.

Hanenkrath J, Park JH, Bay C (2025). Training, use, and modifications related to artificial intelligence in postgraduate orthodontic programs in North America. Am J Orthod Dentofac Orthop Off Publ Am Assoc Orthod Its Const Soc Am Board Orthod; 167(1):89-94.e2.

Haynes SN, Richard DCS, Kubany ES (1995). Content validity in psychological assessment: A functional approach to concepts and methods. Psychol Assess; 7(3):238–47.

Hegde S, Nanayakkara S, Jordan A, Jeha O, Patel U, Luu V, et al (2025). Attitudes and Perceptions of Australian Dentists and Dental Students Towards Applications of Artificial Intelligence in Dentistry: A Survey. Eur J Dent Educ; 29(1):9–18.

Hou D, Capote R, Bayirli B, Chan DCN, Huang G (2020). The effect of digital diagnostic setups on orthodontic treatment planning. Am J Orthod Dentofacial Orthop; 157(4):542–9.

Hou S, Zhou T, Liu Y, Dang P, Lu H, Shi H (2023). Teeth U-Net: A segmentation model of dental panoramic X-ray images for context semantics and contrast enhancement. Comput Biol Med; 152:106296.

Hung K, Yeung AWK, Tanaka R, Bornstein MM (2020). Current Applications, Opportunities, and Limitations of AI for 3D Imaging in Dental Research and Practice. Int J Environ Res Public Health; 17(12):4424.

Hwang JJ, Lee J-H, Han S-S, Kim YH, Jeong H-G, Choi YJ, et al (2017). Strut analysis for osteoporosis detection model using dental panoramic radiography. Dentomaxillofacial Radiol; 46(7):20170006.

Jagtap R, Bayrakdar IS, Orhan K, editors (2023). Artificial Intelligence in Temporomandibular Joint Disorders. Artif. Intell. Dent., Cham: Springer International Publishing; [cited 2025 Mar 30]. p. 187–202. Available from: https://link.springer.com/10.1007/978-3-031-43827-1.

Jaju, PP, Bayrakdar IS, Jaju S, Shah V, Orhan K, Jagtap R, editors (2023). Applications of Artificial Intelligence in Dentistry. Artif. Intell. Dent., Cham: Springer International Publishing; [cited 2025 Feb 28]. p. 43–63. Available from: https://link.springer.com/10.1007/978-3-031-43827-1.

Jeong H, Han S-S, Jung H-I, Lee W, Jeon KJ (2024). Perceptions and attitudes of dental students and dentists in South Korea toward artificial intelligence: a subgroup analysis based on professional seniority. BMC Med Educ; 24(1):430.

Jiang J, Wang Z, Zhang Y, Yu X, Guo X, Liu Y (2016). Recent Advances in Orthodontic Archwire Bending Robot System. Recent Pat Mech Eng; 9(2):125–35.

Jiang J, Zhang Y, Wei C, He T, Liu Y (2015). A Review on Robot in Prosthodontics and Orthodontics. Adv Mech Eng; 7(1):198748.

Jorge F, Carolina F, Pedro F (2019). Artificial intelligence in orthodontics. APOS Trends Orthod; 9(4):201–5.

Juneja M, Garg P, Kaur R, Manocha P, Prateek, Batra S, et al (2021). A review on cephalometric landmark detection techniques. Biomed Signal Process Control; 66:102486.

Katyal D, Balakrishnan N (2022). Evaluation of the accuracy and reliability of WebCeph – An artificial intelligence-based online software. APOS Trends Orthod; 12(4):271–6.

Kau CH, Olim S, Nguyen JT (2011). The Future of Orthodontic Diagnostic Records. Semin Orthod; 17(1):39–45.

Kazem BI, Ghaib NH, Grama NMH (2010). Experimental Investigation and Neural Network Modeling for Force System of Retraction T-Spring for Orthodontic Treatment. J Med Devices; 4(2):021001.

Kazimierczak N, Kazimierczak W, Serafin Z, Nowicki P, Nożewski J, Janiszewska-Olszowska J (2024). AI in Orthodontics: Revolutionizing Diagnostics and Treatment Planning—A Comprehensive Review. J Clin Med; 13(2):344.

Kelly CJ, Karthikesalingam A, Suleyman M, Corrado G, King D (2019). Key challenges for delivering clinical impact with artificial intelligence. BMC Med; 17(1):195.

Khalifa M, Albadawy M, Iqbal U (2024). Advancing clinical decision support: The role of artificial intelligence across six domains. Comput Methods Programs Biomed Update; 5:100142.

khan B, Fatima H, Qureshi A, Kumar S, Hanan A, Hussain J, et al (2023). Drawbacks of Artificial Intelligence and Their Potential Solutions in the Healthcare Sector. Biomed Mater Devices ; 1(2):731–8.

Khan MI, Sm L, Gopal T, Neela PK (2022). Artificial intelligence and 3D printing technology in orthodontics: future and scope. AIMS Biophys; 9(3):182–97.

Khanagar Sanjeev B., Al-Ehaideb A, Vishwanathaiah S, Maganur PC, Patil S, Naik S, et al (2021a). Scope and performance of artificial intelligence technology in orthodontic diagnosis, treatment planning, and clinical decision-making - A systematic review. J Dent Sci; 16(1):482–92.

Khanagar Sanjeev B., Al-ehaideb A, Maganur PC, Vishwanathaiah S, Patil S, Baeshen HA, et al (2021b). Developments, application, and performance of artificial intelligence in dentistry – A systematic review. J Dent Sci; 16(1):508–22.

Khanagar Sanjeev B, Alkathiri M, Alyami K, Alhejazi M (2021c). Knowledge, attitudes, and perceptions of dental students towards artificial intelligence in Riyadh, Saudi Arabia. Med Sci; 25(114):1857–67.

Kharroubi SA, Tannir I, Abu El Hassan R, Ballout R (2024). Knowledge, Attitude, and Practices toward Artificial Intelligence among University Students in Lebanon. Educ Sci; 14(8):863.

Kim CS, Samaniego CS, Sousa Melo SL, Brachvogel WA, Baskaran K, Rulli D (2023). Artificial intelligence (A.I.) in dental curricula: Ethics and responsible integration. J Dent Educ; 87(11):1570–3.

Kim H, Shim E, Park J, Kim Y-J, Lee U, Kim Y (2020). Web-based fully automated cephalometric analysis by deep learning. Comput Methods Programs Biomed; 194:105513.

Kim S-Y, Shin Y-S, Jung H-D, Hwang C-J, Baik H-S, Cha J-Y (2018). Precision and trueness of dental models manufactured with different 3-dimensional printing techniques. Am J Orthod Dentofacial Orthop; 153(1):144–53.

Ko C-C, Tanikawa C, Wu T-H, Pastewait M, Jackson CB, Kwon JJ, et al (2019). Machine learning in orthodontics: application review. Embrac Nov Technol Dent Orthod; 1001:117.

Kök H, Acilar AM, İzgi MS (2019). Usage and comparison of artificial intelligence algorithms for determination of growth and development by cervical vertebrae stages in orthodontics. Prog Orthod; 20(1):41.

Krois J, Ekert T, Meinhold L, Golla T, Kharbot B, Wittemeier A, et al (2019). Deep Learning for the Radiographic Detection of Periodontal Bone Loss. Sci Rep; 9(1):8495.

Krois J, Garcia Cantu A, Chaurasia A, Patil R, Chaudhari PK, Gaudin R, et al (2021). Generalizability of deep learning models for dental image analysis. Sci Rep; 11(1):6102.

Kulikowski CA (1980). Artificial intelligence methods and systems for medical consultation. IEEE Trans Pattern Anal Mach Intell; PAMI-2(5):464–76.

Kunz F, Stellzig-Eisenhauer A, Zeman F, Boldt J (2020). Artificial intelligence in orthodontics : Evaluation of a fully automated cephalometric analysis using a customized convolutional neural network. J Orofac Orthop Fortschritte Kieferorthopadie OrganOfficial J Dtsch Ges Kieferorthopadie; 81(1):52–68.

Kuwada C, Ariji Y, Kise Y, Funakoshi T, Fukuda M, Kuwada T, et al (2021). Detection and classification of unilateral cleft alveolus with and without cleft palate on panoramic radiographs using a deep learning system. Sci Rep; 11(1):16044.

Lagravère MO, Flores-mir C (2005). The treatment effects of Invisalign orthodontic aligners: A systematic review. J Am Dent Assoc; 136(12):1724–9.

Larkin A, Kim J -S., Kim N, Baek S -H., Yamada S, Park K, et al (2024). Accuracy of artificial intelligence-assisted growth prediction in skeletal Class I preadolescent patients using serial lateral cephalograms for a 2-year growth interval. Orthod Craniofac Res; 27(4):535–43.

Lawshe CH (1975). A QUANTITATIVE APPROACH TO CONTENT VALIDITY[1]. Pers Psychol; 28(4):563–75.

Lee K, Torkfar G, Fraser C (2015a). An Investigation into Orthodontic Clinical Record Taking. Int J Orthod Milwaukee Wis; 26(3):53–7.

Lee K-Y, Cho J-W, Chang N-Y, Chae J-M, Kang K-H, Kim S-C, et al (2015b). Accuracy of three-dimensional printing for manufacturing replica teeth. Korean J Orthod; 45(5):217.

Lee Jeong-Hoon, Yu H-J, Kim M, Kim J-W, Choi J (2020a). Automated cephalometric landmark detection with confidence regions using Bayesian convolutional neural networks. BMC Oral Health; 20(1):270.

Lee Jeong-Hee, Han S-S, Kim YH, Lee C, Kim I (2020b). Application of a fully deep convolutional neural network to the automation of tooth segmentation on panoramic radiographs. Oral Surg Oral Med Oral Pathol Oral Radiol; 129(6):635–42

Lee Ki-Sun, Ryu J-J, Jang HS, Lee D-Y, Jung S-K (2020c). Deep Convolutional Neural Networks Based Analysis of Cephalometric Radiographs for Differential Diagnosis of Orthognathic Surgery Indications. Appl Sci; 10(6):2124.

Lee K.S., Kwak HJ, Oh JM, Jha N, Kim YJ, Kim W, et al (2020d). Automated Detection of TMJ Osteoarthritis Based on Artificial Intelligence. J Dent Res; 99(12):1363–7.

Lestrel PE (1989). Some approaches toward the mathematical modeling of the craniofacial complex. J Craniofac Genet Dev Biol; 9(1):77–91.

Li P, Kong D, Tang T, Su D, Yang P, Wang H, et al (2019). Orthodontic Treatment Planning based on Artificial Neural Networks. Sci Rep; 9(1):2037.

Lin L, Tang B, Cao L, Yan J, Zhao T, Hua F, et al (2023). The knowledge, experience, and attitude on artificial intelligence-assisted cephalometric analysis: Survey of orthodontists and orthodontic students. Am J Orthod Dentofac Orthop Off Publ Am Assoc Orthod Its Const Soc Am Board Orthod; 164(4):e97–e105.

Litsas G, Ari-Demirkaya A (2010). Growth indicators in orthodontic patients. Part 1: comparison of cervical vertebral maturation and hand-wrist skeletal maturation. Eur J Paediatr Dent; 11(4):171–5.

Liu J, Chen Y, Li S, Zhao Z, Wu Z (2021). Machine learning in orthodontics: Challenges and perspectives. Adv Clin Exp Med; 30(10):1065–74.

Liu J, Zhang C, Shan Z (2023). Application of Artificial Intelligence in Orthodontics: Current State and Future Perspectives. Healthcare; 11(20):2760.

Lu C-H, Ko EW-C, Liu L (2009). Improving the video imaging prediction of postsurgical facial profiles with an artificial neural network. J Dent Sci; 4(3):118–29.

Ludlow JB, Gubler M, Cevidanes L, Mol A (2009). Precision of cephalometric landmark identification: Cone-beam computed tomography vs conventional cephalometric views. Am J Orthod Dentofacial Orthop; 136(3):312.e1-312.e10.

Lynn MR (1986). Determination and Quantification Of Content Validity: Nurs Res; 35(6):382???386.

Maestre-Ferrín L, Carrillo-García C, Galán-Gil S, Peñarrocha-Diago María, Peñarrocha-Diago Miguel (2011). Prevalence, Location, and Size of Maxillary Sinus Septa: Panoramic Radiograph Versus Computed Tomography Scan. J Oral Maxillofac Surg; 69(2):507–11.

Makaremi M, Lacaule C, Mohammad-Djafari A (2019). Deep Learning and Artificial Intelligence for the Determination of the Cervical Vertebra Maturation Degree from Lateral Radiography. Entropy; 21(12):1222.

Malik OH, McMullin A, Waring DT (2013). Invisible orthodontics part 1: invisalign. Dent Update; 40(3):203–15.

Martina R, Teti R, D'Addona D, Iodice G. (2006) - Neural network based system for decision making support in orthodontic extractions. In: Pham DT, Eldukhri EE, Soroka AJ, editors. Intell. Prod. Mach. Syst., Oxford: Elsevier Science Ltd; [cited 2025 Feb 28].p.235–40. Available from: https://www.sciencedirect.com/science/article/pii/B9780080451572500456.

Martins HMG (2021). Liability implications of artificial inteligence use in health : fault and risk in public sector healthcare . M.Sc. thesis. Portuguese Catholic University. Portugal.

Martorelli M, Gerbino S, Giudice M, Ausiello P (2013). A comparison between customized clear and removable orthodontic appliances manufactured using RP and CNC techniques. Dent Mater ;29(2):e1–e10.

Masuwai A, Zulkifli H, Hamzah MI (2024). Evaluation of content validity and face validity of secondary school Islamic education teacher self-assessment instrument. Cogent Educ; 11(1):2308410.

McHugh ML (2012). Interrater reliability: the kappa statistic. Biochem Medica; 22(3): 276–82.

McNamara Jr JA (2000). Ordinary Orthodontics: Starting with the End in Mind. World J Orthod; 1(1):45-54

Mehta J (1993). Orthodontic records: why? What? When? & how? Funct Orthod; 10(1):44–51.

Mengi A, Singh RP, Mengi N, Kalgotra S, Singh A (2024). A questionnaire study regarding knowledge, attitude and usage of artificial intelligence and machine learning by the orthodontic fraternity of Northern India. J Oral Biol Craniofacial Res; 14(5):500–6.

Mennella C, Maniscalco U, De Pietro G, Esposito M (2024). Ethical and regulatory challenges of AI technologies in healthcare: A narrative review. Heliyon; 10(4):e26297.

Meriç P, Naoumova J (2020). Web-based Fully Automated Cephalometric Analysis: Comparisons between App-aided, Computerized, and Manual Tracings. Turk J Orthod; 33(3):142–9.

Miragall MF, Knoedler S, Kauke-Navarro M, Saadoun R, Grabenhorst A, Grill FD, et al (2023). Face the Future—Artificial Intelligence in Oral and Maxillofacial Surgery. J Clin Med; 12(21):6843.

Miranda F, Barone S, Gillot M, Baquero B, Anchling L, Hutin N, et al (2023a). Artificial Intelligence Applications in Orthodontics. J Calif Dent Assoc; 51(1):2195585.

Miranda F, Choudhari V, Barone S, Anchling L, Hutin N, Gurgel M, et al (2023b). Interpretable artificial intelligence for classification of alveolar bone defect in patients with cleft lip and palate. Sci Rep; 13(1):15861.

Moghimi S, Talebi M, Parisay I (2012). Design and implementation of a hybrid genetic algorithm and artificial neural network system for predicting the sizes of unerupted canines and premolars. Eur J Orthod; 34(4):480–6.

Mohammad-Rahimi H, Nadimi M, Rohban MH, Shamsoddin E, Lee VY, Motamedian SR (2021). Machine learning and orthodontics, current trends and the future opportunities: A scoping review. Am J Orthod Dentofacial Orthop; 160(2):170–92.

Mohd Tahir N, Wan Hassan WN, Saub R (2019). Comparing retainers constructed on conventional stone models and on 3D printed models: a randomized crossover clinical study. Eur J Orthod; 41(4):370–80.

Monill-González A, Rovira-Calatayud L, d'Oliveira NG, Ustrell-Torrent JM (2021). Artificial intelligence in orthodontics: Where are we now? A scoping review. Orthod Craniofac Res; 24 Suppl 2:6–15.

Murali S, Bagewadi A, S LK, Fernandes A, T J, Panwar A, et al (2023). Knowledge, attitude, and perception of dentists regarding the role of Artificial Intelligence and its applications in Oral Medicine and Radiology: a cross sectional study. J Oral Med Oral Surg; 29(2):22.

Nanda SB, Kalha AS, Jena AK, Bhatia V, Mishra S (2015). Artificial neural network (ANN) modeling and analysis for the prediction of change in the lip curvature following extraction and non-extraction orthodontic treatment. J Dent Spec; 3(2):217.

Nauwelaers N, Matthews H, Fan Y, Croquet B, Hoskens H, Mahdi S, et al (2021). Exploring palatal and dental shape variation with 3D shape analysis and geometric deep learning. Orthod Craniofac Res; 24(S2):134–43.

Navlani M, Makhija PG (2013). Evaluation of skeletal and dental maturity indicators and assessment of cervical vertebral maturation stages by height/width ratio of third cervical vertebra. J Pierre Fauchard Acad India Sect; 27(3):73–80.

Nishimoto S, Sotsuka Y, Kawai K, Ishise H, Kakibuchi M (2019). Personal Computer-Based Cephalometric Landmark Detection With Deep Learning, Using Cephalograms on the Internet. J Craniofac Surg; 30(1):91.

Nunnally JC, Bernstein IH (1994). Psychometric theory 3rd ed., New York: McGraw-Hill ,1994, xxiv+752 pp. Appl Psychol Meas. P.303-5.

Oluwatayo J. A (2012). Validity and reliability issues in educational research. J Educ Soc Res; 2(2):391-400.

Orhan K, Bayrakdar IS, Ezhov M, Kravtsov A, Özyürek T (2020). Evaluation of artificial intelligence for detecting periapical pathosis on cone-beam computed tomography scans. Int Endod J; 53(5):680–9.

Orhan K, Jagtap R (2023). Introduction to Artificial Intelligence. In: Orhan K, Jagtap R, editors. Artif. Intell. Dent., Cham: Springer International Publishing; [cited 2025 Feb 28]. p. 1–7. Available from: https://doi.org/10.1007/978-3-031-43827-1_1.

Palanivel J, D D, Srinivasan D, N.C. SC, Kalidass P, Kishore S, et al (2021). Artificial Intelligence – Creating the Future in Orthodontics – A Review. J Evol Med Dent Sci; 10(28):2108–13.

Paredes V, Gandia JL, Cibrián R (2006). Digital diagnosis records in orthodontics. An overview. Med Oral Patol Oral Cirugia Bucal; 11(1):E88-93.

Park J-H, Hwang H-W, Moon J-H, Yu Y, Kim H, Her S-B, et al (2019). Automated identification of cephalometric landmarks: Part 1—Comparisons between the latest deep-learning methods YOLOV3 and SSD. Angle Orthod; 89(6):903–9.

Park JH, Kim Y-J, Kim Jaehyun, Kim Jinie, Kim I-H, Kim N, et al (2021). Use of artificial intelligence to predict outcomes of nonextraction treatment of Class II malocclusions. Semin Orthod; 27(2):87–95.

Park WJ, Park J-B (2018). History and application of artificial neural networks in dentistry. Eur J Dent; 12(04):594–601.

Patcas R, Bernini DAJ, Volokitin A, Agustsson E, Rothe R, Timofte R. (2019). Applying artificial intelligence to assess the impact of orthognathic treatment on facial attractiveness and estimated age. Int J Oral Maxillofac Surg; 48(1):77–83.

Pethani F (2021). Promises and perils of artificial intelligence in dentistry. Aust Dent J; 66(2):124–35.

Polit DF, Beck CT (2004). Nursing research: Principles and methods. Lippincott Williams & Wilkins; [cited 2025 Feb 22]. Available from: https://books.google.com/books?hl=en&lr=&id=5g6VttYWnjUC&oi=fnd&pg=PA3&dq=Polit,+D.F.+and+Beck,+C.T.+(2004)+Nursing+Research:+Principles+and+Methods.+Lippincott+Williams+and+Wilkins,+Philadelphia,+PA,+7th+edn.&ots=_1kLqIloxH&sig=8I3uEmw7kqM8hTUX_ytQRr1fWNY.

Polit DF, Beck CT, Owen SV (2007). Is the CVI an acceptable indicator of content validity? Appraisal and recommendations. Res Nurs Health; 30(4):459–67.

Pringle AJ, Kumaran V, Missier MS, Nadar ASP (2024). Perceptiveness and Attitude on the use of Artificial Intelligence (AI) in Dentistry among Dentists and Non-Dentists - A Regional Survey. J Pharm Bioallied Sci; 16(Suppl2):S1481–S1486.

Promberger M, Baron J (2006). Do patients trust computers? J Behav Decis Mak; 19(5):455–68.

Rahimi B, Nadri H, Lotfnezhad Afshar H, Timpka T (2018). A Systematic Review of the Technology Acceptance Model in Health Informatics. Appl Clin Inform; 09(03):604–34.

Rajpurkar P, Irvin J, Ball RL, Zhu K, Yang B, Mehta H, et al (2018). Deep learning for chest radiograph diagnosis: A retrospective comparison of the CheXNeXt algorithm to practicing radiologists. PLOS Med; 15(11):e1002686.

Ramesh AN, Kambhampati C, Monson JRT, Drew PJ (2004). Artificial intelligence in medicine. Ann R Coll Surg Engl; 86(5):334–8.

Retrouvey J-M, Abdallah M-N, editors (2021). 3D Diagnosis and Treatment Planning in Orthodontics: An Atlas for the Clinician. 1st ed. Cham: Springer International

Publishing;[cited 2025 Feb 27]. Available from: https://link.springer.com/10.1007/978-3-030-57223-5.

Retrouvey J-M, Panayi N, Tsolakis A, editors (2021a). Evolution of the Orthodontic Diagnosis in the Age of Artificial Intelligence. 3D Diagn. Treat. Plan. Orthod. Atlas Clin. 1st ed., Cham: Springer International Publishing; [cited 2025 Jan 10]. p. 3–18. Available from: https://link.springer.com/10.1007/978-3-030-57223-5.

Retrouvey J-M, Vandersluis YR, Kaku J, Vasudavan S, editors (2021b). Three-dimensional treatment simulations for predictable orthodontic treatment planning and implementation. 3D Diagn. Treat. Plan. Orthod. Atlas Clin. 1st ed., Cham: Springer International Publishing; [cited 2025 Feb 27]. p. 239–64. Available from: https://link.springer.com/10.1007/978-3-030-57223-5.

Roganović J, Radenković M, Miličić B (2023). Responsible Use of Artificial Intelligence in Dentistry: Survey on Dentists' and Final-Year Undergraduates' Perspectives. Healthcare; 11(10):1480.

Rokaya D, Jaghsi AA, Jagtap R, Srimaneepong V (2024). Artificial intelligence in dentistry and dental biomaterials. Front Dent Med; 5:1525505.

Salmi M, Tuomi J, Sirkkanen R, Ingman T, Mäkitie A (2012). Rapid Tooling Method for Soft Customized Removable Oral Appliances. Open Dent J; 6:85–9.

Samad N, Noor MAM, Mansor M, Jumahat T (2023). Measuring the Content Validity of Middle Leadership Competence Model using Content Validity Ratio (CVR) Analysis. Int J Bus Technol Manag; 5(4):134–44.

Sangoseni O, Hellman M, Hill C (2013). Development and Validation of a Questionnaire to Assess the Effect of Online Learning on Behaviors, Attitudes, and Clinical Practices of Physical Therapists in the United States Regarding Evidenced-based Clinical Practice. Internet J Allied Health Sci Pract; 11(2):1-12

Scheideman GB, Bell WH, Legan HL, Finn RA, Reisch JS (1980). Cephalometric analysis of dentofacial normals. Am J Orthod; 78(4):404–20.

Schultz KS, Whitney DJ (2005). Measurement theory in action: Case studies and Exercises.2455 Teller Road, Thousand Oaks California 91320 United States:SAGE Publications, Inc. P.436.

Schwendicke F, Golla T, Dreher M, Krois J (2019). Convolutional neural networks for dental image diagnostics: A scoping review. J Dent; 91:103226.

Schwendicke F, Rossi JG, Göstemeyer G, Elhennawy K, Cantu AG, Gaudin R, et al (2021). Cost-effectiveness of Artificial Intelligence for Proximal Caries Detection. J Dent Res; 100(4):369–76.

Schwendicke F, Samek W, Krois J (2020). Artificial Intelligence in Dentistry: Chances and Challenges. J Dent Res; 99(7):769–74.

Seram T, Batra M, Gijwani D, Chauhan K, Jaggi M, Kumari N (2021). Attitude and perception of dental students towards artificial intelligence. Univ J Dent Sci; 7(3):77-81

Shafi S, Khan FA, Umar D, Shetty S, Koya S, Devadasan DD (2024). Artificial Intelligence in Orthodontics: A Thorough Assessment of its Influence and Applications. Int J Oral Care Res; 12(1):31.

Shan T, Tay FR, Gu L (2021). Application of Artificial Intelligence in Dentistry. J Dent Res; 100(3):232–44.

Sherman SL, Kadioglu O, Currier GF, Kierl JP, Li J (2020). Accuracy of digital light processing printing of 3-dimensional dental models. Am J Orthod Dentofacial Orthop; 157(3):422–8.

Shoukri B, Prieto JC, Ruellas A, Yatabe M, Sugai J, Styner M, et al (2019). Minimally Invasive Approach for Diagnosing TMJ Osteoarthritis. J Dent Res; 98(10):1103–11.

Steiner CC (1953). Cephalometrics for you and me. Am J Orthod, St Louis; 39(10):729-55

Strunga M, Urban R, Surovková J, Thurzo A (2023). Artificial Intelligence Systems Assisting in the Assessment of the Course and Retention of Orthodontic Treatment. Healthcare; 11(5):683.

Subramanian AK, Chen Y, Almalki A, Sivamurthy G, Kafle D (2022). Cephalometric Analysis in Orthodontics Using Artificial Intelligence—A Comprehensive Review. BioMed Res Int; 2022(1):1880113.

Surendran A, Daigavane P, Shrivastav S, Kamble R, Sanchla AD, Bharti L, et al (2024). The Future of Orthodontics: Deep Learning Technologies. Cureus; 16(6);e62045.

TaherdoostP H (2018). A review of technology acceptance and adoption models and theories. Procedia Manuf; 22:960–7.

Tahir K, Abul Barakaat ,Afeefa, Fida ,Mubassar, and Sukhia RH (2024). In the Contemporary Era of Artificial Intelligence, the Trajectory of Orthodontics: Past and Future Perspectives – A Narrative Review. J Calif Dent Assoc; 52(1):2400420.

Takada K (2016). Artificial intelligence expert systems with neural network machine learning may assist decision-making for extractions in orthodontic treatment planning. J Evid-Based Dent Pract; 16(3):190–2.

Tamer İ, Öztaş E, Marşan G (2019). Orthodontic Treatment with Clear Aligners and The Scientific Reality Behind Their Marketing: A Literature Review. Turk J Orthod; 32(4):241–6.

Terry DA, Snow SR, McLaren EA (2008). CE 1-contemporary dental photography: selection and application. Compendium; 29(8):432.

Thanathornwong B (2018). Bayesian-Based Decision Support System for Assessing the Needs for Orthodontic Treatment. Healthc Inform Res; 24(1):22.

Thorat V, Rao P, Joshi N, Talreja P, Shetty AR (2024). Role of Artificial Intelligence (AI) in Patient Education and Communication in Dentistry. Cureus; 16(5):e59799.

Thurzo A, Kurilová V, Varga I (2021). Artificial Intelligence in Orthodontic Smart Application for Treatment Coaching and Its Impact on Clinical Performance of Patients Monitored with AI-TeleHealth System. Healthc Basel Switz; 9(12):1695.

Tilden VP, Nelson CA, May BA (1990). Use of Qualitative Methods to Enhance Content Validity. Nurs Res; 39(3):172.

Tomášik J, Zsoldos M, Oravcová Ľ, Lifková M, Pavleová G, Strunga M, et al (2024). AI and Face-Driven Orthodontics: A Scoping Review of Digital Advances in Diagnosis and Treatment Planning. AI; 5(1):158–76.

Topol EJ (2019). High-performance medicine: the convergence of human and artificial intelligence. Nat Med; 25(1):44–56.

Tsolakis AI, Kalavritinos M, Bitsanis E, Sanoudos M, Benetou V, Alexiou K, et al (2018). Reliability of different radiographic methods for the localization of displaced maxillary canines. Am J Orthod Dentofacial Orthop; 153(2):308–14.

Tsolakis IA, Kolokitha O-E, Papadopoulou E, Tsolakis AI, Kilipiris EG, Palomo JM (2022). Artificial Intelligence as an Aid in CBCT Airway Analysis: A Systematic Review. Life; 12(11):1894.

Tsui WK, Chua HDP, Cheung LK (2012). Bone anchor systems for orthodontic application: a systematic review. Int J Oral Maxillofac Surg; 41(11):1427–38.

Vaishnavi D, Sheethal J, Kishore K (2021). Robotic Wire Bending in Orthodontics .Dentistry; 11(5):1-3.

Vandenberghe B, Jacobs R, Bosmans H (2010). Modern dental imaging: a review of the current technology and clinical applications in dental practice. Eur Radiol; 20(11):2637–55.

Waltz CF (2005). Measurement in Nursing and Health Research. 3rd ed. New York, NY: Springer Publishing Company. P.201-45

Waltz CF, Strickland OL, Lenz ER (1991). Measurement in nursing research. Philadelphia: F.A. Davis Co. 2nd ed; [cited 2025 Feb 22]. Available from: https://cir.nii.ac.jp/crid/1130000796047730688.

Waltz CF, Strickland OL, Lenz ER (2005). Measurement in nursing and health research. 3rd ed. New York , NY: Springer Publishing Company. P.201-45

Wang X, Pastewait M, Wu T-H, Lian C, Tejera B, Lee Y-T, et al (2021). 3D morphometric quantification of maxillae and defects for patients with unilateral cleft palate via deep learning-based CBCT image auto-segmentation. Orthod Craniofac Res; 24(S2):108–16.

Wei G, Cui Z, Liu Y, Chen N, Chen R, Li G, et al (2020). TANet: Towards Fully Automatic Tooth Arrangement. In: Vedaldi A, Bischof H, Brox T, Frahm J-M, editors. Comput. Vis. – ECCV 2020, Cham: Springer International Publishing; p. 481–97.

Weir T (2017). Clear aligners in orthodontic treatment. Aust Dent J; 62(S1):58–62.

Williamson YM (1981). Research methodology and its application to nursing. New York: Wiley. P.325.

Wilson FR, Pan W, Schumsky DA (2012). Recalculation of the Critical Values for Lawshe's Content Validity Ratio. Meas Eval Couns Dev; 45(3):197–210.

Wong KF, Lam XY, Jiang Y, Yeung AWK, Lin Y (2023). Artificial intelligence in orthodontics and orthognathic surgery: a bibliometric analysis of the 100 most-cited articles. Head Face Med; 19(1):38.

Wu M-J, Zhao K, Fils-Aime F (2022). Response rates of online surveys in published research: A meta-analysis. Comput Hum Behav Rep; 7:100206.

Xiao Z, Liu Z, Gu Y (2020). Integration of digital maxillary dental casts with 3D facial images in orthodontic patients. Angle Orthod; 90(3):397–404.

Xie X, Wang L, Wang A (2010). Artificial Neural Network Modeling for Deciding if Extractions Are Necessary Prior to Orthodontic Treatment. Angle Orthod; 80(2):262–6.

Yagi M, Ohno H, Takada K (2010). Decision-making system for orthodontic treatment planning based on direct implementation of expertise knowledge. Annu Int Conf IEEE Eng Med Biol Soc IEEE Eng Med Biol Soc Annu Int Conf; 2010:2894–7.

Yassir YA, McIntyre GT, Bearn DR (2016). Three questionnaires to assess the perception of fixed orthodontic therapy before, during and after treatment: validity and reliability. Eur J Orthod; 39(4):402-410.

Yassir YA, Salman AR, Nabbat SA (2022). The accuracy and reliability of WebCeph for cephalometric analysis. J Taibah Univ Med Sci; 17(1):57–66.

Yongde Z, Chunge W, Jingang J, Jixiong J, Yi L, Yong W (2014). Motion Planning for Archwire Bending Robot in Orthodontic Treatments. Int J Control Autom; 7(7):287–98.

Yu AC, Mohajer B, Eng J (2022). External Validation of Deep Learning Algorithms for Radiologic Diagnosis: A Systematic Review. Radiol Artif Intell; 4(3):e210064.

Yu HJ, Cho SR, Kim MJ, Kim WH, Kim JW, Choi J (2020). Automated Skeletal Classification with Lateral Cephalometry Based on Artificial Intelligence. J Dent Res; 99(3):249–56.

Yüzbaşıoğlu E (2021). Attitudes and perceptions of dental students towards artificial intelligence. J Dent Educ; 85(1):60–8.

Zhao JY, Song B, Anand E, Schwartz D, Panesar M, Jackson GP, et al (2017). Barriers, Facilitators, and Solutions to Optimal Patient Portal and Personal Health Record Use: A Systematic Review of the Literature. AMIA Annu Symp Proc AMIA Symp; 2017:1913–22.

Zhao T, Zhou J, Yan J, Cao L, Cao Y, Hua F, et al (2021). Automated Adenoid Hypertrophy Assessment with Lateral Cephalometry in Children Based on Artificial Intelligence. Diagnostics; 11(8):1386.

Appendix I

The content validity assessment form included the invitation letter and the initial draft of the survey items

A) Cover letter

Invitation letter to Contribute to Dental AI Research Questionnaire **Content Validity Assessment**

Title

Perception, Attitudes, and Application of Dental Artificial Intelligence Among Iraqi Orthodontists

Researcher:

Dr. Noor Nadheer Al-Taie

MSc Candidate (Orthodontics)

Hawler Medical University /College of Dentistry

noor.altaie@den.hmu.edu.krd

Supervisor:

Assist. Prof. Dr. Shaho Ziyad Al-Talabani

BDS., MSc., PhD (Orthodontics)

Hawler Medical University/College of Dentistry

shaho.talabani@hmu.edu.krd

Confidentiality Notice:

Your participation is voluntary, and your response will be kept confidential. The feedback you provide will be used solely to validate the content of the final questionnaire.

Thank you in advance for your consideration and potential contribution to this research. I look forward to your response, and I am available to answer any questions you may have.

B) Content validation section

Dear Doctor,

As part of the study, we intend **to validate** the questionnaire items that have been developed.

Purpose of the questionnaire: -

The questionnaire focuses on understanding Iraqi Orthodontists' scientific knowledge, awareness, and attitudes toward using dental artificial intelligence in their clinical practice.

Given your expertise in orthodontics, I would like to invite you to join the **Content validity experts panel** to gather **Evidence-Based items** for potential Inclusion in the final questionnaire.

Your valuable input will help ensure the survey instrument **includes all the essential items** and **eliminates undesirable items** related to a particular construct domain.

If you are willing to contribute, I kindly ask you **to assess the level of importance of** each item/question in the questionnaire as:-

- Either — Essential
- Or — Useful but Not Essential
- Or — Not necessary

Note: Please review each question and write your rating **by marking the appropriate column** with **X** using the **(Instrument Rating Form)** below

C) Instrument rating sheet

Instrument Rating Form

Kindly review **each question** in each section below and rate it by simply typing an **X** into the appropriate column of the relevant question.

Elements	(Check only ONE for each row)			Comments if you have/Suggestions, or Recommendations
Section 1: Demographic data and professional background	Essential	**Useful, but NOT essential**	NOT Necessary	
Q1				
Q2				
Q3				
Q4				
Q5				
Q6				
Section 2: Knowledge and awareness				
Q 1				
Q 2				
Q 3				
Section 3: Perception about the Use of AI in Orthodontic Practice	Essential	**Useful, but NOT essential**	NOT Necessary	Your Recommendations
Q 1				
Q 2				
Q 3				
Q 4				
Section 4: Attitudes about the Use of AI in Orthodontics	Essential	**Useful, but NOT essential**	NOT Necessary	Your Recommendations
Q 1				
Q 2				
Q 3				
Q 4				
Q 5				
Q 6				
Q 7				
Q 8				
Section 5: Impact of Dental AI in Orthodontic Practice	Essential	**Useful, but NOT essential**	NOT Necessary	Your Recommendations
Q 1				
Q 2				
Q 3				
Section 6: Challenges, Limitations, and Future of AI in Orthodontics	Essential	**Useful, but NOT essential**	NOT Necessary	Your Recommendations
Q 1				
Q 2				
Q 3				
Q 4				
Q 5				

D) Survey questions original draft

Survey Questionnaire

1. **<u>Demographic data and professional background</u>**

Q1) What is your gender?

- ○ Female ○ Male

Q2) How old are you?

- ○ <30 years
- ○ 30-40 years
- ○ >40 years

Q3) What is your academic achievement?

- ○ M.Sc. in Orthodontics
- ○ PhD in Orthodontics

Q4) How many years of clinical experience do you have?

- ○ < 5 years
- ○ 5-10 years
- ○ >10 years

Q5) Which institution do you belong to?

- ○ Ministry of Health
- ○ Ministry of higher education and scientific research
- ○ Others

Q6) What is your main region of residency?

- ○ Northern region of Iraq
- ○ Central region of Iraq
- ○ Southern region of Iraq
- ○ Eastern region of Iraq
- ○ Western region of Iraq

2. Knowledge and awareness of AI

Q1) How did you hear about AI applications certainly designed for orthodontics?[Select all that apply]

- ○ Social media (Facebook, Instagram, Twitter)
- ○ Professional education (Courses, Conferences, Lectures at the university)
- ○ Family and Colleagues
- ○ Scientific journals and books
- ○ I have not obtained any information from any source

Q2) How would you evaluate your scientific knowledge about AI in orthodontics?

○ Basic ○ Intermediate ○ Advanced ○ Expert

Q3) Which AI Orthodontic software have you used? [Select all that apply]

- ○ Bluesky
- ○ Webceph
- ○ NEMOFAB
- ○ RayFace
- ○ Progressive orthodontic simulation app
- ○ Others
- ○ I have not used any AI Software program

3. **Perception about the use of AI in Orthodontic practice**

Q1) Are you aware of the use of AI-powered software programs for diagnosis and treatment planning in orthodontic practice?

O Yes O No

Q2) Are you aware of the utilization of AI in digitization and lateral cephalometric analysis?

O Yes O No

Q3) Are you aware of AI's role in preparing and planning for orthognathic surgery/Correcting facial aesthetics?

O Yes O No

Q4) In your opinion, is the diagnosis and treatment planning of AI-powered software is better than that of an experienced human orthodontist?

O Yes O No O Maybe

4. **Attitudes about the use of AI in Orthodontics**

Q1) Are you currently using AI-powered tools in your orthodontic practice?

O Never O Rarely O Often O Always

Q2) Which type of activity do you use AI for in your practice?[Select all that apply]

O Diagnosis

O Treatment planning

O Patient's education and communication

O Practice management

O I don't use AI in my clinical practice

Q3) If the clinical decision and artificial intelligence's decision differ, which one do you trust?

O Orthodontist's decision O AI's decision O Not sure

Q4) Are you aware of the utilization of AI-assisted tools like the prediction of canine impaction, determination of the geometry of orthodontic spring with force to align the teeth, and software to select the suitable headgear?

○ Yes ○ No

Q5) In which area of orthodontics do you think AI will be promising? [Select all that apply]

○ Diagnosis

○ Treatment planning

○ Performance of CBCT analysis and lateral cephalometric analysis with simulation

○ Space analysis

○ Bracket positioning

○ Determining biomechanics of orthodontic treatment

○ Clear aligner treatment

○ VTO [Visual treatment objective for Dental arches]

○ VTO [Visual treatment objective for facial changes]

○ Direct treatment using AI-assisted robots (e.g. Insertion guide for MARPE)

Q6) Do you find that AI-assisted orthodontics saves the time for diagnosis and treatment planning?

○ Yes ○ No ○ Maybe

Q7) Do you agree that AI-assisted orthodontics will boost treatment costs?

○ Yes ○ No ○ Maybe

Q8) Would you be interested in receiving formal training on AI in orthodontics and integrating AI-based tools in your practice?

○ Yes ○ No

5. Impact of Dental AI in orthodontic practice

Q1) How has AI impacted your clinical decision-making process during orthodontic diagnosis and treatment planning?

- ○ Significantly improved
- ○ Somewhat improved
- ○ No impact
- ○ Somewhat decreased
- ○ Significantly decreased

Q2) Rate the impact of dental AI on the following **aspects** of orthodontics

	Negative	**Neutral**	**Positive**
Efficiency in orthodontic diagnosis and treatment planning			
Accuracy in orthodontic diagnosis and treatment planning			
Patient Experience			

Q3)Do you agree that the use of AI would improve the treatment quality and accuracy in orthodontics?

○ Strongly disagree ○ Disagree ○ Neutral ○ Agree ○ Strongly agree

6. Challenges, limitations, and future of AI in orthodontics

Q1) What do you think are the biggest challenges in adopting AI in Orthodontics? [Select all that apply]

- ○ High Cost of creation and design
- ○ Humans become less driven and inactive
- ○ Lack of training
- ○ Concerns about accuracy and effectiveness
- ○ Data privacy
- ○ Trust in technology
- ○ Lack of regulatory policies that govern AI use in Dentistry

Q2) Do you believe artificial intelligence could substitute orthodontists in clinical practice?

○ Yes ○ No ○ Maybe

Q3) Do you believe orthodontists can base on AI-powered programs as a second judgment in complex cases for diagnosis and treatment in the near future?

○ Yes ○ No ○ Maybe

Q4) Do you think AI will play a significant role in the future of orthodontic practice in Iraq?

○ Yes ○ No ○ Unsure

Q5) Do you believe AI-related education training should be included in undergraduate and postgraduate orthodontic curriculum?

○ Yes ○ No

Appendix II

The invitation letter, face validity assessment form, and the survey questions draft after content validation.

A) Cover letter

Invitation letter to Contribute to Dental AI Research Questionnaire **Face Validity Assessment**

Title

Perception, Attitudes, and Application of Dental Artificial Intelligence Among Iraqi Orthodontists

Researcher:

Dr. Noor Nadheer Al-Taie

BDS., MSc Candidate (Orthodontics)

Hawler Medical University /College of Dentistry

noor.altaie@den.hmu.edu.krd

Supervisor:

Assist. Prof. Dr. Shaho Ziyad Al-Talabani

BDS., MSc., PhD (Orthodontics)

Hawler Medical University/College of Dentistry

shaho.talabani@hmu.edu.krd

Confidentiality Notice:

Your participation is voluntary, and your response will be kept confidential. The feedback you provide will be used solely to improve and refine the questionnaire items.

Thank you in advance for your consideration, time, support, and potential contribution to this research. I look forward to your response, and I am available to answer any questions you may have.

B) Face validation section

Dear Doctor,

As part of this research study, we seek expert input to ensure the clarity and consistency of these survey items through the face validation process.

Purpose of the questionnaire: - This questionnaire focuses on understanding Iraqi Orthodontists' scientific knowledge, awareness, and attitudes toward using dental artificial intelligence in their clinical practice.

Given your expertise in the clinical and educational fields of orthodontics, I would like to invite you to join the face validity expert panel and assess the survey items based on the following seven criteria:

1)Consistency and relevance of items to the survey's perceived goal.

2) Suitability of the layout.

3)Appropriateness of language difficulty concerning the respondents' level of knowledge.

4)Proper text font size and line spacing.

5)Spelling accuracy of complex terms.

6)The transparency and clear meaning of items.

7)Accurate and suitable grammatical usage.

Your expertise and valuable insights will greatly enhance the quality and validity of the survey items, ensuring they are feasible, readable, well-formatted, stylistically appropriate, and evident in language.

If you are willing to participate, please review the survey questions in the attached copy of this letter, and for each criterion, rate the survey items as either:

Yes (Indicating the questions meet the relevant criterion)

Or

No (Indicating no agreement or need for revision)

Furthermore, we would appreciate any suggestions, comments, and recommendations for further improvement and refinement of the questionnaire items.

C) Face validity rating form

Face Validity Rating Form

Kindly review all the survey questions, and for each of the following criteria, indicate your rating by simply typing either Yes or No in the corresponding row.

Assessment criteria	Expert rating **either** (Yes or **No**)
1) Consistency and relevance of items to the survey's perceived goal.	
2) Suitability of the layout.	
3)Appropriateness of language difficulty concerning the respondents' level of knowledge	
4)Proper text font size and line spacing	
5)Spelling accuracy of complex terms.	
6)The transparency and clear meaning of items	
7)Accurate and suitable grammatical usage.	

D) Further perspectives, comments, and suggestions

<u>Your comments, suggestions, and recommendations</u>

E) Survey questions following content validation

Survey questionnaire sections and questions

1. **Demographic data and professional background**

Q1) What is your gender?

○ Female ○ Male

Q2) What is your (Year) of birth?

……………………………………………………………………..

Q3) What is your academic achievement?

○ M.Sc. in Orthodontics
○ PhD in Orthodontics

Q4) How many years of clinical experience do you have in orthodontics?

○ < 5 years
○ 5-10 years
○ >10 years

Q5) Which institution do you belong to?

○ Ministry of Health
○ Ministry of higher education and scientific research
○ Others

Q6) What is your main region of residency?

○ Northern region of Iraq
○ Central region of Iraq
○ Southern region of Iraq
○ Eastern region of Iraq
○ Western region of Iraq

2. Knowledge and awareness of AI

Q1) How did you learn about AI software programs specifically designed for orthodontics? [Select all that apply]

- ○ Social media (Facebook, Instagram, Twitter)
- ○ Web browsing (Google advertisements, Internet Explorer, YouTube advertisements, ……etc.)
- ○ Professional education (courses, conferences, lectures at the university)
- ○ Family and Colleagues
- ○ Scientific journals and books
- ○ I have not obtained any information from any source

Q2) Which AI orthodontic software have you used? [Select all that apply]

- ○ Bluesky
- ○ Webceph
- ○ NEMOFAB
- ○ RayFace
- ○ Progressive orthodontic simulation app
- ○ Others
- ○ I have not used any AI software program

Q3) Are you aware of using AI-powered software programs for diagnosis and treatment planning in orthodontic practice?

○ Yes ○ No

Q4) Are you aware of the use of AI in digitization and lateral cephalometric analysis?

○ Yes ○ No

Q5) Are you aware of AI's role in the preparation and planning of orthognathic surgery or in correcting facial aesthetics

O Yes O No

Q6) Are you aware of using AI-assisted tools like the prediction of canine impaction, determination of the geometry of orthodontic spring with force to align the teeth, and software to select the suitable headgear?

O Yes O No

3. Perception about the use of AI in Orthodontic practice

Q1) Do you find that AI-assisted orthodontics saves time for diagnosis and treatment planning?

O Yes O No O Maybe

Q2) If the clinical decision differs from the artificial intelligence decision, which one do you trust?

O Orthodontist's decision O AI's decision O Not sure

Q3) In your opinion, is the diagnosis and treatment planning of AI-powered software is better than that of an experienced human orthodontist?

O Yes O No O Maybe

4. Attitudes about the use of AI in Orthodontics

Q1) Are you currently using AI-powered tools in your orthodontic practice?

○ Never ○ Rarely ○ Often ○ Always

Q2) In which area of orthodontics would you apply AI if its results prove to be promising? [Select all that apply]

- ○ Diagnosis
- ○ Treatment planning
- ○ CBCT analysis and lateral cephalometric analysis with simulation
- ○ Space analysis
- ○ Bracket positioning
- ○ Determination of the biomechanics of orthodontic treatment
- ○ Clear aligner treatment
- ○ VTO [Visual treatment objective for dental arches]
- ○ VTO [Visual treatment objective for facial changes]
- ○ Direct treatment using AI-assisted robots (e.g. Insertion guide for MARPE)
- ○ Practice management
- ○ Patient's education and communication

Q3) Would you be interested in receiving formal training on AI in orthodontics and integrating AI-based tools into your practice?

○ Yes ○ No

5. Impact of Dental AI in orthodontic practice

Q1) How has AI impacted your clinical decision-making process during orthodontic diagnosis and treatment planning?

- ○ Significantly improved
- ○ Somewhat improved
- ○ No impact
- ○ Somewhat decreased
- ○ Significantly decreased

Q2) Rate the impact of dental AI on the following **aspects** of orthodontics.

	Negative	**Neutral**	**Positive**
Efficiency in orthodontic diagnosis and treatment planning			
Accuracy in orthodontic diagnosis and treatment planning			
Patient Experience			

Q3) Do you agree that the use of AI can improve the treatment quality and accuracy in orthodontics?

○ Strongly disagree ○ Disagree ○ Neutral ○ Agree ○ Strongly agree.

6. The Challenges, limitations, and future of AI in orthodontics

Q1) What do you think are the biggest challenges in adopting AI in Orthodontics? [Select all that apply]

- ◯ High Cost of creation and design
- ◯ Humans become less driven and inactive
- ◯ Lack of training
- ◯ Concerns about accuracy and effectiveness
- ◯ Data privacy
- ◯ Trust in technology
- ◯ Lack of regulatory policies that govern AI use in Dentistry

Q2) Do you believe artificial intelligence could substitute orthodontists in clinical practice?

◯ Yes ◯ No ◯ Maybe

Q3) Do you believe orthodontists could rely on AI-powered programs as a secondary tool for judgment in complex cases for diagnosis and treatment planning in the near future?

◯ Yes ◯ No ◯ Maybe

Q4) Do you think AI will play a significant role in the future of orthodontic practice in Iraq?

◯ Yes ◯ No ◯ Unsure

Q5) Do you recommend including AI-related education training in undergraduate and postgraduate orthodontic curricula?

◯ Yes ◯ No

Appendix III

Survey sections and questions after content and face validation.

1. Demographic data and professional background

Q1) What is your gender?

○ Female ○ Male

Q2) What is your (Year) of birth?

....

Q3) What is your highest academic qualification?

○ M.Sc. in Orthodontics

○ PhD in Orthodontics

Q4) How many years of clinical experience do you have in orthodontics?

○ < 5 years

○ 5-10 years

○ >10 years

Q5) Which institution are you affiliated with?

○ Ministry of Health

○ Ministry of higher education and scientific research

○ Others

Q6) What is your region of residence?

○ Northern region of Iraq

○ Central region of Iraq

○ Southern region of Iraq

○ Eastern region of Iraq

○ Western region of Iraq

2. Knowledge and awareness of AI

Q1) How did you learn about AI software programs specifically designed for orthodontics? [Select all that apply.]

- ○ Social media (Facebook, Instagram, Twitter)
- ○ Web browsing (Google advertisements, Internet Explorer, YouTube advertisements, etc.)
- ○ Professional education (courses, conferences, lectures at the university)
- ○ Family and Colleagues
- ○ Scientific journals and books
- ○ I have not obtained any information from any source

Q2) Which AI orthodontic software have you used? [Select all that apply.]

- ○ Bluesky
- ○ Webceph
- ○ NEMOFAB
- ○ RayFace
- ○ Progressive orthodontic simulation app
- ○ Others
- ○ I have not used any AI software program

Q3) Are you aware of using AI-powered software programs for diagnosis and treatment planning in orthodontic practice?

○ Yes ○ No

Q4) Are you aware of the use of AI in digitization and lateral cephalometric analysis?

○ Yes ○ No

Q5) Are you aware of AI's role in the preparation and planning of orthognathic surgery or in correcting facial aesthetics?

○ Yes ○ No

Q6) Are you familiar with using AI-assisted tools, such as predicting canine impaction, determining the geometry of orthodontic springs used to apply force for teeth alignment, and software for selecting the appropriate headgear?

○ Yes ○ No

3. <u>Perception about the use of AI in Orthodontic practice</u>

Q1) Do you believe that AI-assisted orthodontics helps save diagnosis and treatment planning time?

○ Yes ○ No ○ Maybe

Q2) If the clinical decision differs from the artificial intelligence decision, which one do you trust?

○ Orthodontist's decision ○ AI's decision ○ Not sure

Q3) Do you believe the diagnosis and treatment planning provided by AI-powered software are superior to those of an experienced orthodontist?

○ Yes ○ No ○ Maybe

4. Attitudes about the use of AI in Orthodontics

Q1) Are you currently using AI-powered tools in your orthodontic practice?

○ Never ○ Rarely ○ Often ○ Always

Q2) In which area of orthodontics would you apply AI if its results prove to be promising? [Select all that apply]

○ Diagnosis

○ Treatment planning

○ CBCT analysis and lateral cephalometric analysis with simulation

○ Space analysis

○ Bracket positioning

○ Determination of the biomechanics of orthodontic treatment

○ Clear aligner treatment

○ VTO [Visual treatment objective for dental arches]

○ VTO [Visual treatment objective for facial changes]

○ Direct treatment using AI-assisted robots (e.g. Insertion guide for MARPE)

○ Practice management

○ Patient's education and communication

Q3) Would you be interested in receiving formal training on AI in orthodontics and integrating AI-based tools into your practice?

○ Yes ○ No

5. Impact of Dental AI in orthodontic practice

Q1) To what extent has AI impacted your clinical decision-making process during orthodontic diagnosis and treatment planning?

- ○ Significantly improved
- ○ Somewhat improved
- ○ No impact
- ○ Somewhat decreased
- ○ Significantly decreased

Q2) Rate the impact of dental AI on the following **aspects** of orthodontics.

	Negative	**Neutral**	**Positive**
Efficiency in orthodontic diagnosis and treatment planning			
Accuracy in orthodontic diagnosis and treatment planning			
Patient Experience			

Q3) Do you agree that the use of AI can improve the treatment quality and accuracy in orthodontics?

○ Strongly disagree ○ Disagree ○ Neutral ○ Agree ○ Strongly agree.

6. The Challenges, limitations, and future of AI in orthodontics

Q1) What do you consider to be the biggest challenges in adopting AI in orthodontics? [Select all that apply]

- ○ High Cost of creation and design
- ○ Humans become less driven and inactive
- ○ Lack of training
- ○ Concerns about accuracy and effectiveness
- ○ Data privacy
- ○ Trust in technology
- ○ Lack of regulatory policies that govern AI use in Dentistry

Q2) Do you believe artificial intelligence could substitute orthodontists in clinical practice?

○ Yes ○ No ○ Maybe

Q3) Do you believe orthodontists could rely on AI-powered programs as a secondary tool for judgment in complex cases for diagnosis and treatment planning in the near future?

○ Yes ○ No ○ Maybe

Q4) Do you think AI will play a significant role in the future of orthodontic practice in Iraq?

○ Yes ○ No ○ Unsure

Q5) Do you recommend including AI-related education training in undergraduate and postgraduate orthodontic curricula?

○ Yes ○ No

FSC
www.fsc.org
MIX
Papier | Fördert gute Waldnutzung
FSC® C083411

Kolibri 360 GmbH
Ferdinand-Jühlke-Straße 7
99095 Erfurt, Deutschland
produktsicherheit@kolibri360.de

Druck:
CPI Druckdienstleistungen GmbH
im Auftrag der
Kolibri 360 GmbH
Ferdinand-Jühlke-Str. 7
99095 Erfurt